THE *Healthy* ALTERNATIVE

Why Chiropractic Care Is the Safest and Most Effective Way to Restore and Maintain Optimal Health...Naturally!

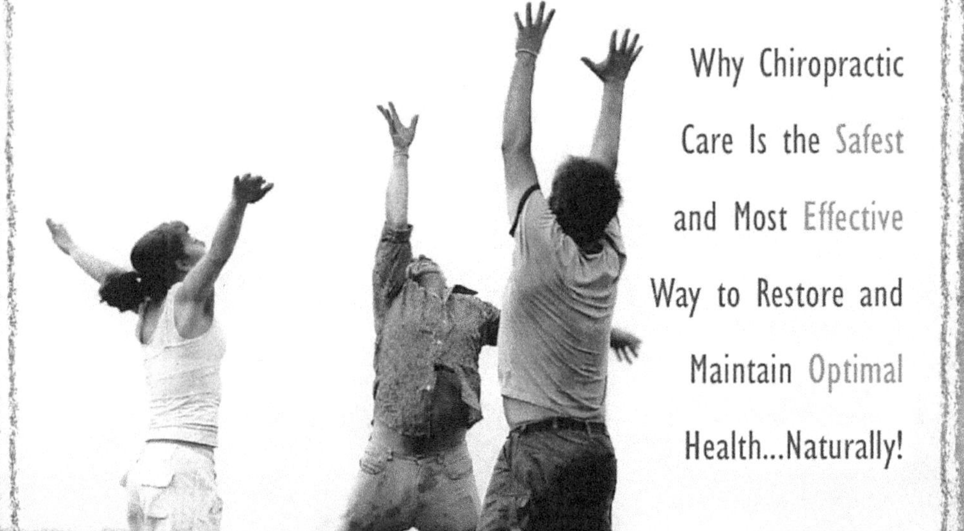

Dr. Michael & Dr. Torri Gambacorta

The Healthy alternative

Why Chiropractic is the Safest and
Most Effective Way to Restore and Maintain
Optimal Health... Naturally

THANK YOU FOR TAKING
AN INTEREST IN YOUR
Health, AND FOR
READING OUR BOOK.
Sincerely yours in Health,
Dr. Mike Gambacorta

Thank you for choosing
us! We look forward
to helping you in
the future
Dr Torri Gambacorta

TABLE OF CONTENTS:

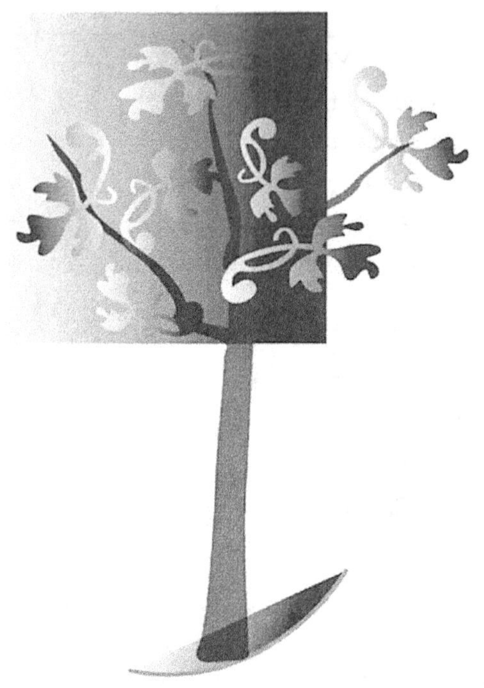

So, What Exactly Are Your Alternatives?

OKAY, PLEASE RAISE your hand if you like living with daily pain... or if you want to grow old and not be able to do the things you enjoy...

My bet is you're not raising your hand right now -- and not just because you're reading a book and you'd look a little nutty if you were!

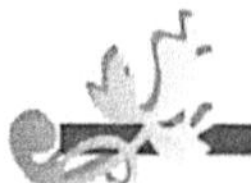

Nobody wants to live with pain and certainly nobody wants to grow old -- when growing old means giving up the things you love to do and the ability to care for yourself.

But unfortunately the stress and pressures of daily living take a toll on our bodies. There isn't a single person who doesn't experience bouts of aches and pains at some point in his life. The important question is -- what do you do when those aches and pain show up on your doorstep and even more importantly, what do you do to make sure they don't keep coming back! This is your choice to make.

The Pill Popping Alternative

LET'S SAY YOU WERE playing tennis the other week and during your second set you felt something in your elbow "go out." Or perhaps you were digging into some spring-cleaning and realized a moment too late just how heavy that box was you were trying to pick up. The bottom line is you're now in pain. So what are you going to do?

For many people, the answer is simple -- take a painkiller. In fact, if you stop by your neighborhood medical doctor he'll probably offer the same solution. After all, medical doctors are trained to treat ailments in just two primary ways -- medication or surgery. No big secret here.

While drugs and surgery are the appropriate treatment in many cases, and can sometimes even work wonders, they are not always the answer -- especially when it comes to relieving your pain.

The fact of the matter is very few people know the truth about the dangers of "popping pills," and even fewer doctors are willing to admit it!

> *Did you know each year in the United States an estimated 140,000 people die from drug-related reactions?*
>
> *Did you know it is estimated that up to 98,000 Americans die yearly from medical errors -- a doctor accidentally making the wrong incision, a nurse administering the wrong medication, and so on?* [1]
>
> *That's almost one-quarter of a million deaths each year in the United States alone due to the adverse affects of surgery and drug treatment. It's certainly a good reason to pause a moment before running straight to the doctor, isn't it!*

Now back to that aching tennis elbow or stiff lower back. Most drugs used to treat pain fall into one of three categories:

    (1) analgesics that are non-steroidal anti-inflammatories (NSAIDs) or non-narcotic painkillers;

    (2) analgesics that are narcotic painkillers;

    (3) muscle relaxers.

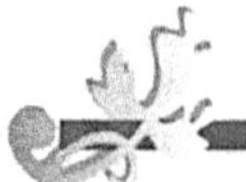

Chapter 1: Healthy and Pain-Free Life

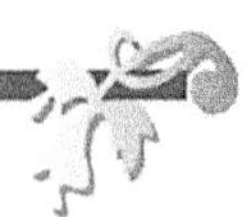

(1)   Let's look first at **analgesics** that are either non-steroidal anti-inflammatories or non-narcotic painkillers. Analgesics are a class of drug used to reduce pain by either blocking pain signals sent to your brain or by interfering with your brain's interpretation of those signals.

You're probably familiar with non-steroidal anti-inflammatory drugs, or NSAIDs for short, and other non-narcotic painkillers by their more common brand names: Tylenol, Bayer, Ecotrin, Advil, Motrin, Nuprin, Aleve, Naprosyn, Anaprox, and Naprelen.

While these medications can be safe – it is only when they are taken

    a) in amounts not exceeding the recommended dosage, and

    b) for a short period of time.

The problem is due to the chronic and often severe nature of many injuries and ailments -- it's impossible to experience lasting relief while sticking to these prescription regulations. Most medical doctors opt to disregard these guidelines.

To make matters worse, your body biochemically adapts to these drugs, and thus you have to take higher and higher dosages to feel the same relief.

You might be wondering,

"What's the big deal about taking a little extra Tylenol for a few weeks or even months? I can buy it at the supermarket, so it can't be dangerous."

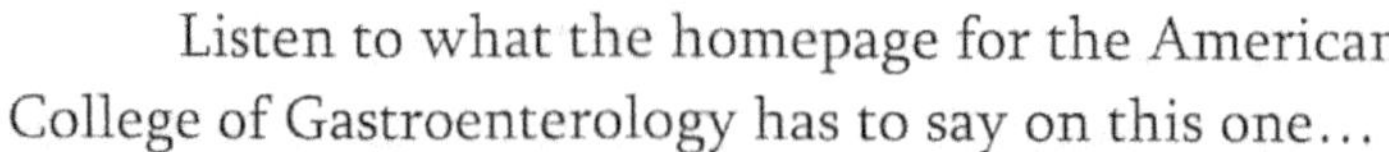

Listen to what the homepage for the American College of Gastroenterology has to say on this one…

"The second major cause for ulcers is irritation of the stomach arising from regular use of non-steroidal anti-inflammatory drugs, or NSAIDs. NSAIDs are available over-the-counter (OTC) and by prescription."

So what exactly is a peptic ulcer? That's the official medical name.

It's a sore on the lining of your stomach -- not much different than a regular sore except it's on your inside.

So how do NSAIDs cause ulcers?

Well, as a child, did you ever wonder why your stomach doesn't digest itself? Your body makes strong acids that are used to break down the food you eat. There's a special lining that protects your stomach from these harsh acids.

What happens when you take a couple of little red and white Tylenol for your backache?

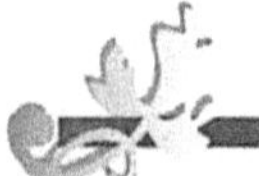

NSAIDs and aspirin break down that special lining, and those harsh acids slowly burn into your stomach. Your stomach begins to eat itself away.

If you have ever experienced even the slightest symptoms of ulcers, you understand how excruciating it is to wake up in the middle of the night with a burning in your stomach or be unable to enjoy a simple meal because of the acid eating away your gut.

And take heed before you have even a glass of water! Drinking water when you suffer from ulcers is like pouring alcohol on an open wound!

You might still be wondering -- isn't this all a little extreme? Taking aspirin and Advil for my aches and pains can't be that dangerous.

A breaking new study unfortunately confirmed that the dangers of NSAIDs are even worse than imagined. Using a new "swallowable, capsule-size camera," researchers at the Baylor College of Medicine were able to view the damage done by NSAIDs in a brand-new light.

The results were shocking.

The videos from the micro-camera showed that 71% of all NSAID users had suffered injury to their small intestine (compared to 5% of non-NSAID-users).

They even did a study with those good ol' red and white friends -- Tylenol. In a group of 40 patients, half took acetaminophen only and the others took nothing at all. The sphincter muscle controls the opening of the

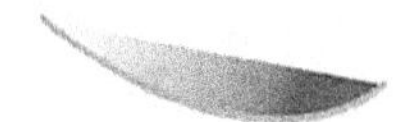

stomach (at the point where the stomach opens to the upper portion of the small intestine). Of the 20 individuals taking acetaminophen, one in four were shown to have suffered severe damage to their small bowel. Not some or partial, but severe damage.

So if your doctor tells you to rest up and just take some Tylenol for your pain, and he advises you to do this for any length of time more than about a week, or if his recommended dosage exceeds the restrictions on the bottle -- don't do it!

You will undoubtedly damage, and possibly severely injure your stomach.

Again -- even the manufacturer admits it on the bottle's label -- these medications are not meant to be taken in large dosages or for extended periods of time.

(2)   What if instead your doctor chooses to prescribe a narcotic painkiller for your aches and pains?

These drugs are different from aspirin and NSAIDs because they are derived from opiates. What does this mean? You guessed it, in addition to the many other health risks, these drugs are also addictive.

You might recognize these substances by their more common names -- perhaps your doctor has even prescribed one for you in the past:

Oxycodone, morphine, codeine, Demerol, oxymorphone, methadone, and others…

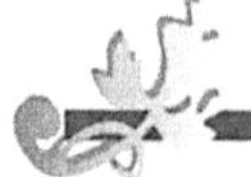

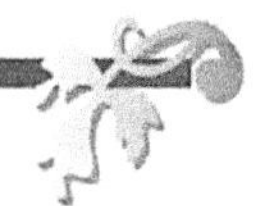

Do these drugs work?

Absolutely -- if your definition of "working" is providing relief from severe or chronic pain.

However, each and every time you take one of these drugs to relieve your pain, your body develops a greater tolerance. For this class of drug to continue working, you are required to take higher and higher doses.

This is the path to dependence and addiction.

The word addiction may conjure images of hoodlums dealing drugs in an alley. While narcotic painkillers are certainly highly popular on the black market, the dependence and addiction we're talking about here is simply the inability to function normally without taking a specific substance.

You probably don't need to think very hard to think of someone you know, a friend, family member or co-worker, who began taking narcotic painkillers for an injury or ailment and now takes them regularly just to get through the day. They may not be a "drug user" in our regular understanding of the word -- but make no mistake, they are addicted.

According to eMedicine,

> *"Some people with intense pain get such high doses that the same dose would be fatal if taken by someone who was not suffering from pain."*

How does that sound for a solution to your back pain? Begin taking a highly addictive substance, continue taking it as your back pain persists, and increase your dosages until you are taking an amount that if you took initially would've killed you?

Remember these drugs which medical doctors prescribe every day with greater and greater frequency are "opioids." They are the same chemical class as heroine.

Whether your doctor prescribes a narcotic or non-narcotic painkiller for your back pain, the critical problem is this… NONE of these medications can actually fix or heal the cause of your pain.

Therefore as your pain persists, if you do not seek other help, you must take these drugs, and in ever-higher dosages to function.

In your quest to be free of back pain, you will inevitably compromise and endanger your short- and long-term health. Period.

(3)   The last item on the "pill popping" menu for relieving your pain are muscle relaxers.

You've probably heard of Flexeril, Soma, and Valium. Maybe you've even tried them to relieve a bad lower back pain or tension headache.

Ever wonder how muscles relaxers really work?

Anesthetists, the doctors who put you to sleep before surgery, use muscle relaxers during an operation to make sure you don't move. Muscle relaxers block the

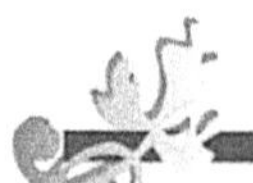

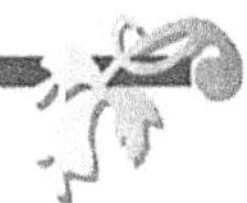

receptors on the muscle. In other words, they prevent your ability to feel pain.

While pain is not enjoyable, it is a healthy function of the body.

When you twist your back the wrong way or you bend to pick up something too heavy, pain tells you to stop because your body is being hurt, injured, or damaged. Without pain, you would be burning your hands on pot handles and cutting yourself with razors without even knowing about it.

While muscle relaxers can certainly be beneficial when used for a little while, let's look at what happens if you take muscle relaxers for a long time.

Say you have a backache, and oh boy is it a doozey. You hate sitting around the house, missing work and not being able to do the things you usually do. But it's just too painful when you try to do these things. So even though you don't like medications, you cave in and decide to take the 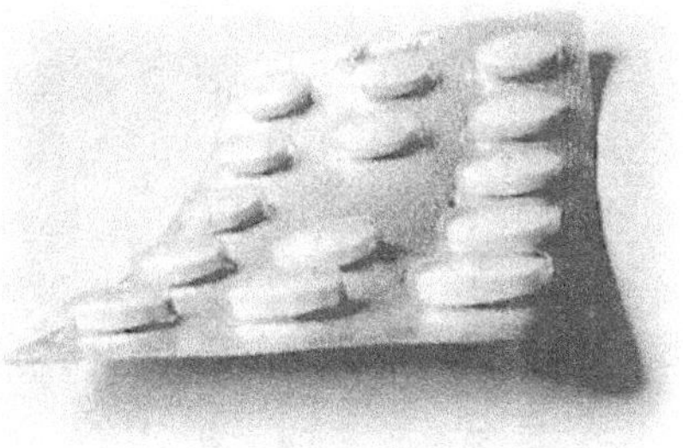 muscle relaxers your family doctor prescribed. Soon you find yourself back in the routine and moving around as the muscle relaxers interfere with your nervous system communication and your pain disappears! Or does it…

Just because you are not experiencing back pain, doesn't mean your back isn't *in pain.* Sure, you feel better for the moment. You go right back to doing all the things that used to make you clutch and wince in agony. You're walking and moving around, stretching and picking up things, maybe you even start hitting the gym again…

Unbeknownst to you, you are creating greater and greater damage to your body and a bigger and bigger back problem every single day.

The reason your body was sending you pain signals when you bent over to pick something up, was because your back was injured and couldn't safely move that way. It's your body's way of saying, *"Please don't bend down like this, we'll hurt our back even more."*

By taking muscle relaxers you've essentially told your body to *"Shut up!"*

Don't be surprised to discover when you stop taking muscle relaxers your back is even more severely injured and you're in even greater pain than before!!

Before we bid adieu to those nasty bottles of pills, there is one last option for pain that's becoming quite the hit amongst medical doctors when it comes to treating back pain. It's not a drug in the sense that it's a pill, but it is a medication.

And if you thought those other drugs were dangerous, hold onto your seat!

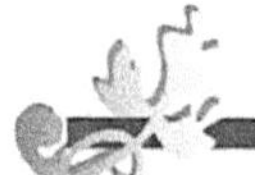

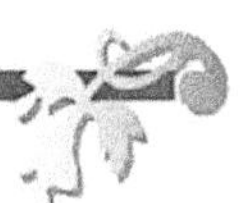

What if your doctor wanted to relieve your back pain by injecting a substance into your back that was not recommended by the Physicians Desk Reference?

What if the manufacturer of this drug even strongly recommended doctors not to do this to you?

What if this injection to relieve your back pain was shown to be improperly administered one out of four times and was the only known cause of an incurable condition described as "sheer hopeless hell"?

And what if your doctor wanted to inject this substance directly into your spine!?!

Welcome to the world of Epidural Steroid Injections -- ESIs for short.

ESIs have become a choice treatment of medical doctors for back pain. If your family doctor ever refers you to a "pain clinic," this is where you're headed.

In a nutshell, in an attempt to reduce back pain and inflammation, pain doctors use an x-ray guided injection of steroids put directly into your spine.

Sound fun?

The Physician's Desk Reference (or PDR), the bible doctors are supposed to follow when prescribing medications, specifically states:

"Suitable sites for intra-articular injection are the knee, ankle, wrist, elbow, shoulder, phalangeal,

*and hip joints... Joints not suitable for injection
are those that are anatomically inaccessible, such
as the spinal joints."*

Again, joints not suitable for injection include spinal joints!

In fact, the manufacturer's label for Depo-Medrol, the product name for this injectable steroid, also specifically warns:

"Joints not suitable for injection are those that are anatomically inaccessible such as the spinal joints..."

Epidural Steroid Injections have even been banned in several countries around the world because insurance companies refuse to cover any doctor who performs these high-risk injections.

So what makes epidural injections so incredibly dangerous?

You don't have to be a brain surgeon to realize injecting a syringe directly into your spine is not a safe or natural way to relieve back pain.

An epidural injection delivers steroids directly into the epidural space in the spine via a very long needle. The epidural space is a thin area between the dura mater, a membrane, and the wall of your vertebrae. While these shots can be highly effective because they reduce inflammation at the very root, that's also what makes them so perilous.

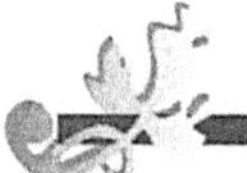

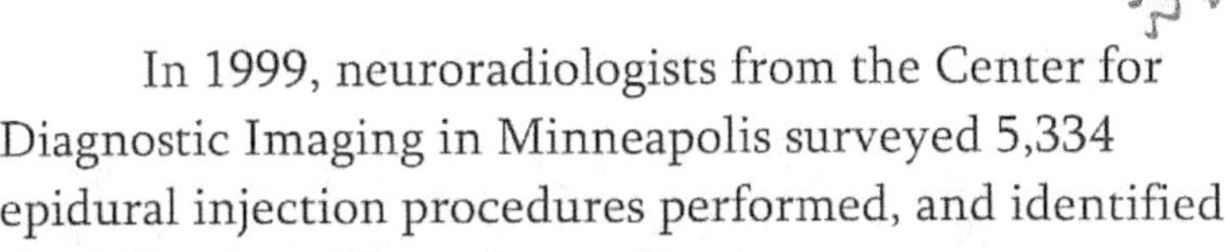

In 1999, neuroradiologists from the Center for Diagnostic Imaging in Minneapolis surveyed 5,334 epidural injection procedures performed, and identified the following risks and complications:

> *"The blind interlaminar technique introduces the potential for erroneous needle placement and subsequent injection of substances into undesired locations, such as the subarachnoid space".*

The authors noted that blind needle injection, even by "skilled and experienced procedurists" has been found to be inaccurate in 25-30% of cases.[2]

Stop the presses!

> *"Blind needle injection, even by 'skilled and experienced procedurists' has been found to be inaccurate in 25-30% of cases"!*

That means if a pain doctor wants to give you just a single epidural injection, just to "see if it helps your back pain," you have a one in four chance of becoming victim of an inaccurate injection. And that's if he's a "skilled and experienced procedurist"!

If he recommends you get one shot a week for the next four weeks or four months to relieve your back pain, statistically you are guaranteed to become victim of an inaccurate blind needle injection to your spine.

So what's the big deal about haphazard, inaccurate injections to your spine?

Certainly the doctor standing at the other end of the needle isn't too worried.

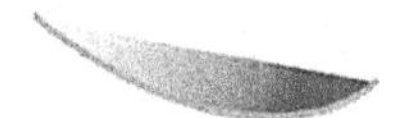

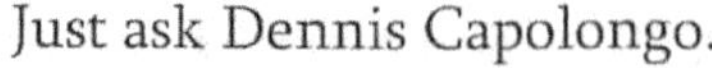

Just ask Dennis Capolongo.

A nagging hip pain prompted Dennis to visit his medical doctor. After receiving just two epidural injections he suffered two trips to the hospital, was hospitalized and suffered non-stop back pain.

That's not even the real tragedy. Dennis developed arachnoiditis -- a pain disorder caused by the inflammation of the arachnoid -- that's one of the membranes that can easily be damaged as a result of blind epidural injections.

He can no longer work or do anything he used to because of his condition.

He describes the condition as "sheer, hopeless hell".

There is no cure.

Dennis invests the little strength he now has to warn unknowing patients like you of the horrific dangers of epidural injections.

Sadly, pain management is a big business and the insurance reimbursement for epidural injections is quite lucrative -- so many pain management centers have become "procedure mills."

The most mind blowing part of this whole tragedy -- there is no proof that Depo-Medrol provides any pain relief at all!

According to the American Society of Health-System Pharmacists:

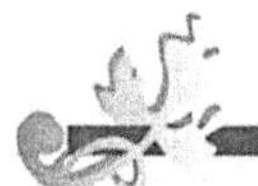

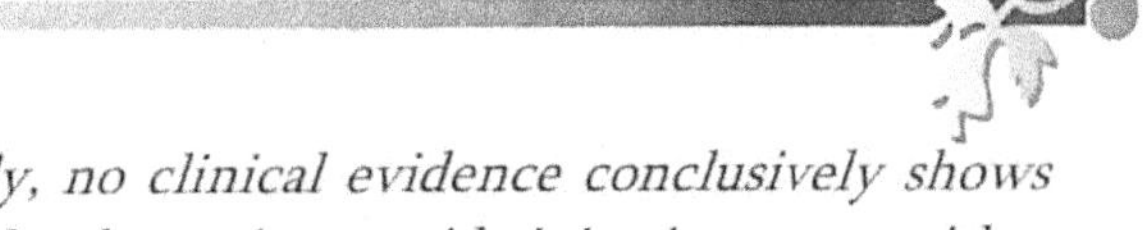

"Currently, no clinical evidence conclusively shows that epidural corticosteroid injections are either effective or ineffective for relieving low back pain." [3]

That's right. With all the risks and damage to your health, doctors who recommend these injections do not even have any clinical evidence that the injections will help you at all!

THE SURGERY ALTERNATIVE

WELL THEN, WHEN IT COMES to your bum knee or bad back, medical doctors still have one more choice of treatment -- to put you under the knife.

Before you jump at this chance, and sticking with backs for the moment, take a peek at these alarming statistics published in the Washington Post Health Section, April 20, 1995:

> *"In this country, surgeons perform more than 250,000 lower back operations annually -- at an average hospital cost of $11,000, excluding surgeon's fees -- and health officials think that much of the surgery is unnecessary."*

You heard right, health officials think much of the surgery is unnecessary!

Just ask Dr. Arthur H. White, internationally renowned orthopedic spine surgeon and recognized leader in the field of spine surgery and rehabilitation, who confessed in this article:

> *"Exploratory surgery to search for the cause of a patient's pain is...useless. You don't operate on a chronic patient unless the pain is intolerable, unless you know for sure that the pain is generated by a specific malfunction in the back, and that surgery has been shown to correct this particular problem. But these rules of thumb are not always followed."*

Again -- for a surgeon to operate without knowing the exact cause of your back pain is useless. Yet there's a good possibility this will happen to you, according to Dr. White.

Dr. White reveals, *"I make my living on cleaning up the messes of other surgeons who have operated prematurely with inadequate diagnosis and inadequate training."*

Not only is back surgery a potentially huge cost for you, but it may also be completely unnecessary and ineffective.

And there is another complication that comes with surgery that few if any doctors will ever take the time to talk about.

William Abdu is an associate professor and director of the Spine Center at Dartmouth Medical College in Hanover, N.H. Dr. Abdu regrettably admits,

> *"We can't make these people normal -- that is, healthy with full function -- and we shouldn't think we can. If any doctor is telling you this -- whether they admit it or not -- they are telling you a lie."*

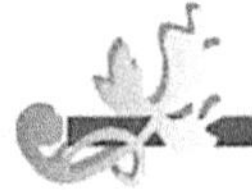

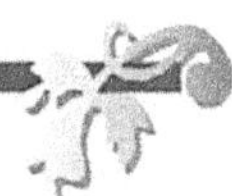

When it comes to serious pain problems the spider effects are so much further-reaching than just the isolated physical cause; it's foolish to think surgery will give you back your "old life."

Just consider the surgery statistics which reveal that for individuals who require surgery, three of every four will not return to work for up to four years because of pain. Ouch!

By now you're probably starting to realize medications and surgery do not provide the pain relief and restoration you need to return to living normally.

The bottom line is medical doctors are not effectively trained to treat pain.

That's why they just prescribe medications or refer you to other specialists who either prescribe harsher medications or recommend surgery.

The most you can hope for is a little bit of relief, but it will not last long.

Now this isn't to say all medical doctors are evil and greedy or out to get you. In fact, most medical doctors really do care. However, they just lack the training to use anything but medications or surgery to treat your ailments.

The "Let Nature Take Its Course" Alternative

MAYBE YOU'RE THINKING with all these crazy medications and surgical procedures, if you suffer an injury or are in pain, your best bet is to just "rest up" till you feel better.

If your medical doctor is bit more on the conservative side, he might even give you this same bit of advice.

Certainly bed rest is good medication and the right first step to recovery -- so long as it only lasts two to three days.

You see, prolonged bed rest can actually make your injury even worse.

Dr. Scott Fishman runs the pain-management program at the University of California, Davis School of Medicine.

He reveals that while years ago doctors recommended bed rest to give patients time to heal, that is absolutely not recommended today.

"In fact, not moving can be the worst medicine."[4]

Moving is essential in order for the joints in your body to flush out toxins, feed themselves, and begin the healing and regeneration process.

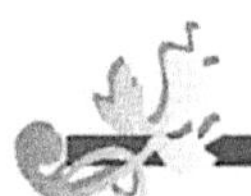

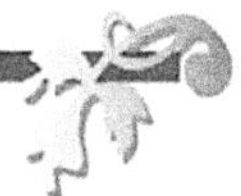

So if you think lying in bed for weeks is your ticket to feeling like new -- think again.

The course of nature on your body is the same as it is on all other matter. Ever hear of entropy and the Second Law of Thermodynamics?

Left alone, all matter moves from order to disorder. Another way to look at it is if no energy is added to or leaves the system, the potential energy will always be less than the initial energy. And the same holds true for our bodies.

> Okay, let me make it simple in case you're not a science nerd. All this means is that the stress and fatigue of life is ultimately destined to wear down our bodies. Unless we actively do something otherwise, our body's natural course is to become weaker and less able as the years go by.

THE CHIROPRACTIC ALTERNATIVE

AT THIS POINT YOU MIGHT be feeling like you don't have much of a choice. Our bodies are set on a crash course to break down over time like an old car, and medications and surgery seem to do more damage than good.

When something's wrong in your body, albeit sickness or an injury, treating pain is only a temporary

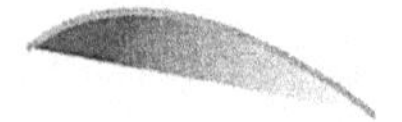

solution. You'll never feel better and whole again until you correct the cause of your problem.

Well, before you start feeling all glum, it's time for the good news -- in fact, it's great news.

> *What if there was a treatment that could correct the root cause of your aches and pains without any risks and restore your body to normal health?*
>
> *What if this remedy was completely natural and even increased your longevity?*
>
> *What if it allowed you to combat the aging process and feel younger and stronger than you have in years?*

You're about to discover all this and much more as you learn about a treatment that has withstood the test of time for thousands of years and is recognized as the safest form of care available anywhere!

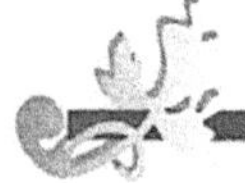

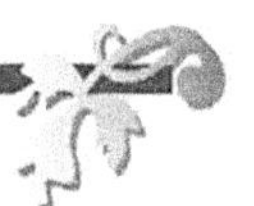

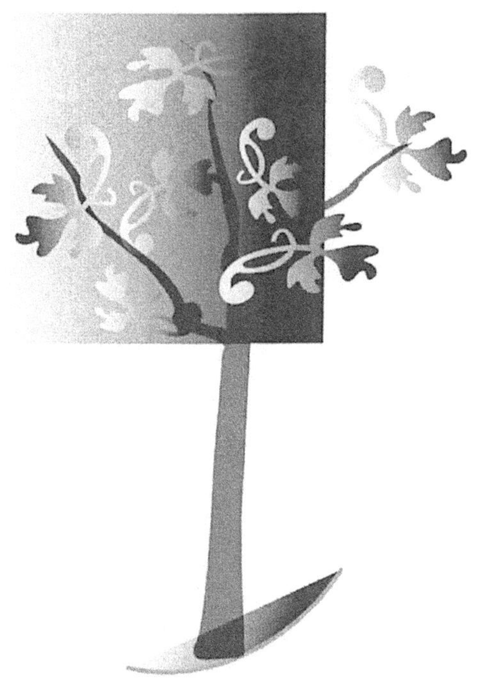

What Exactly Is Chiropractic Care, Anyway?

ASK MOST PEOPLE what a chiropractor does, and they will most likely say, *"He's the guy who cracks your back."* Now ask a chiropractor the same question. He or she will probably say something like, *"A chiropractor reduces spinal subluxations, which allows the body to achieve a state of optimal health."*

CHAPTER
2

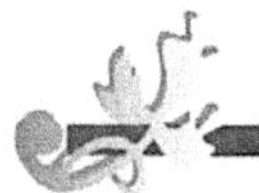

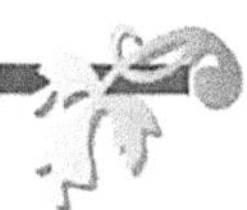

Well, both of those statements are true to a certain degree, but neither statement gives you a clear picture of chiropractic care. Yes, a chiropractor certainly does manipulate the spine (fine, go ahead and call it cracking if you must!), and reducing subluxations -- don't worry, we'll tell you what those are later -- does improve overall health.

But what is chiropractic, really?

Is it an art?

Is it a science?

Actually, it's a little of both, with some philosophy thrown in just to keep things really interesting!

CHIROPRACTIC IS A SCIENCE

CHIROPRACTIC IS A SCIENCE focused mainly on the spine and central nervous system. And there are certain scientific principles that chiropractic follows:

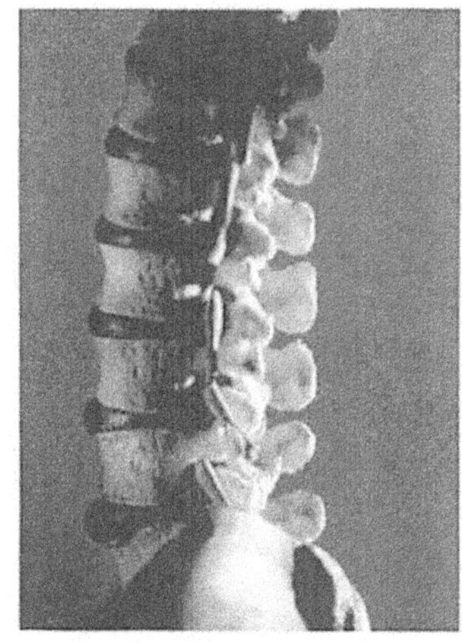

- ♣ diagnoses are made through testing and empirical observations
- ♣ treatment is based on the chiropractor's training and experience.

However, there is a big difference between the science of traditional medicine, and the science of chiropractic care. While traditional medicine uses drugs-- and sometimes even surgery -- to treat patients, medical doctors are primarily focused on treating symptoms of pain and illness, not the root causes.

Chiropractic care has a completely different, albeit equally scientific, approach.

In a nutshell, chiropractic uses manipulation -- you are probably more familiar with the term adjustments -- of the spine to correct misalignments. Why all the hullaballoo about misalignments? Well, misalignments muddy up the communication between the brain, the nervous system, and the rest of the body. And that's not good! We need that communication to be crystal clear in order to experience optimal health. Once the spine is properly realigned, the nerves can go about doing their job of communicating.

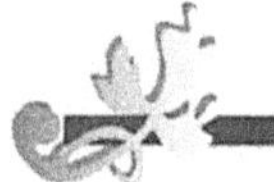

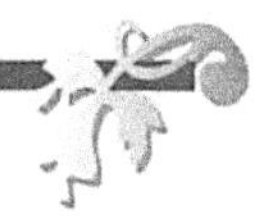

Chiropractic Is An Art

LIKE CONVENTIONAL MEDICINE, chiropractic is an art. But unlike conventional medicine, it is a natural art. That means drugs and surgery are not used. In fact, the goal of chiropractic isn't to heal illness or injury at all, though that does often occur as a rather nice side effect! Rather, the goal is to restore the body to its natural state.

Through the course of our busy lives our bones and soft tissues are misused or overused, and are damaged in the process. A chiropractor is able to manipulate these bones and soft tissues so that they are back in the right place. When they are back in their proper positions, communication between the brain and body can once again resume the way it is supposed to. Once the communication is flowing, the chemical, neurological, and mechanical processes of the body will begin to function properly. When these are functioning properly, your body is able to correct any internal problems and begin healing on its own. It's that simple!

Chiropractic As A Philosophy

CHIROPRACTIC IS ALSO A PHILOSOPHY, one about the causes of life, health, and disease. *Chiropractic believes that our bodies want to express perfect health and well-being, and somewhere inside us our bodies have a certain wisdom that knows how to do this.* Think of

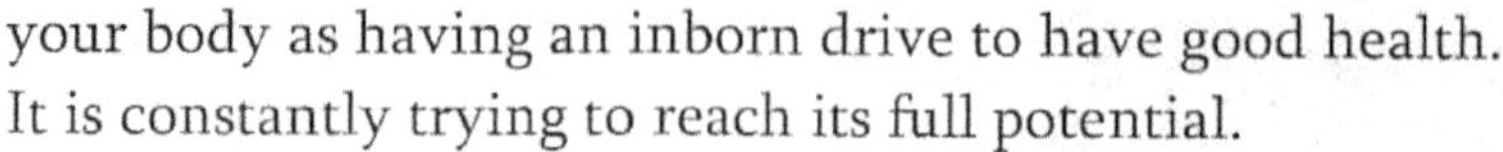

your body as having an inborn drive to have good health. It is constantly trying to reach its full potential.

But sometimes it is not allowed to! Certain physical blocks -- namely bones and soft tissue being out of alignment -- prevent the body from expressing optimal health. The focus of chiropractic is to remove those blocks. Once the blocks are removed, good health is the result.

HISTORY OF CHIROPRACTIC CARE

WHILE YOU MAY THINK chiropractic is a relatively new practice, research shows that people have been adjusting the spine since the beginning of civilization. Ancient Chinese writings show the spine being manipulated as early as 2700 B.C. An ancient writing from Egypt dated 1600 B.C. shows bones being manipulated as well. How else do you think Cleopatra managed to stay healthy despite all that stress? Spinal manipulation was not just confined to one part of the world, either. Societies from the ancient worlds of Babylon, Syria, India, Tibet, and Japan; Native American tribes such as the Sioux, Winnebago, and Creek; and South American groups of Mayan, Aztec, Toltec, Tarascan, and Zoltec Indians -- all used manipulation and adjustment to relieve pain and cure illness.

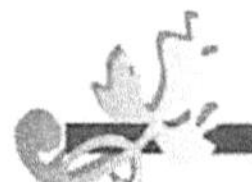

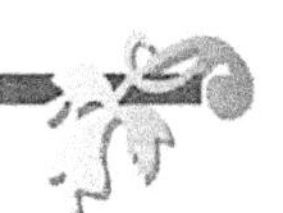

So, how did chiropractic care come to the Western world?

Well, the roots of Western medicine lie in ancient Greece, and start with a man you may have heard of named Hippocrates around 400 B.C. Our friend Hippocrates stirred things up a bit in ancient Greece when he proposed that illnesses and injuries were not a result of the gods being angry. Instead, Hippocrates taught that the human body and the laws of nature were subject to the same forces. Therefore, it was possible for us to have some say in our own health and wellness. We had some control over whether we were sick or well, injured or sound, in pain or pain-free. What a revelation!

In the Hippocratic text *On the Nature of Man*, a healthy body is described as one that is in balance, while an unhealthy body is described as one that is experiencing an imbalance in one of the body's systems. So, what was the job of the ancient Greek physicians?

Well, the first thing they did was encourage healthful living, in order to encourage balance. Think of all the athletes that came out of Greece, and this makes sense! When, inevitably, that balance was disturbed due to illness or injury, the physician would restore that balance. How? Mostly by helping the body heal itself. Instead of focusing on the injury or illness, the physician focused on exercise, diet, manipulation, and rest. Just like today's doctors, ancient physicians were asked, first, to do no harm, and second, to ease symptoms to allow the body

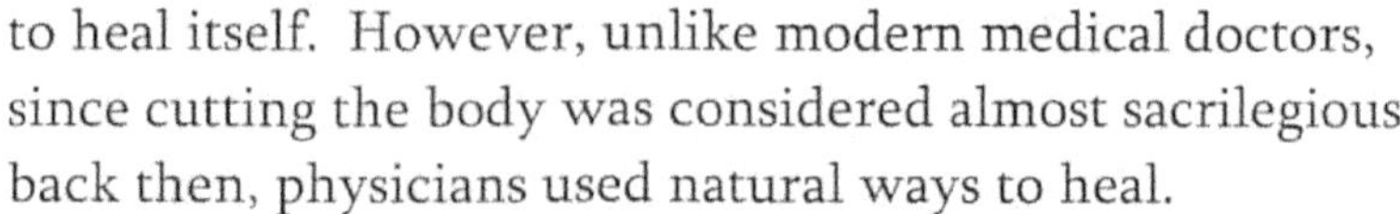

to heal itself. However, unlike modern medical doctors, since cutting the body was considered almost sacrilegious back then, physicians used natural ways to heal.

Several of the works we still have from the Hippocratic school show spinal manipulation as one of the ways to heal. Physicians in the Roman Empire also used the Hippocratic texts to treat illnesses and injury.

All was humming along quite nicely until the fall of the Roman Empire... and the subsequent loss of all that ancient knowledge. Medicine once again became rooted in superstition. While some Islamic physicians and monks continued to treat illnesses in a natural way, for the most part physicians used some very interesting methods to treat their patients. For hundreds of years -- even as late as the eighteenth century -- if you were sick or injured you could look forward to such treatments as purging with laxatives or emetics, bloodletting (draining the body of "bad" blood), or cupping, where scalding hot glasses were placed on the affected areas of the body in an attempt to pull the diseased "humors" out of the body. Ouch! Aren't you glad we have better health care options today?

As they still do today, people had access to unconventional medicine. People who lived in the country especially, far from doctors, turned to folk medicine practitioners. Some of these practitioners were called "bonesetters." Bonesetters fixed broken bones, but they also manipulated the spine and other joints.

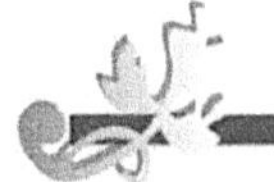

Chapter 2: What Is Chiropractic Care?

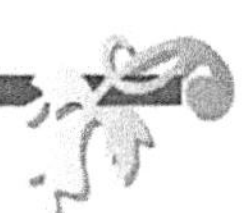

By the nineteenth century, Western medicine had evolved to closely resemble today's medicine. After observing and running tests, doctors would prescribe drugs, or sometimes surgery, in an attempt to alleviate symptoms or cure the disease or injury. Certain physicians, however -- some of whom had even studied with bonesetters -- continued to manipulate the spine and other joints as a part of their treatment.

During the late nineteenth century, two healing practices based on manipulation cropped up. The first of these was osteopathy. *Andrew Taylor Sill*, the father of osteopathy, was a surgeon during the Civil War who was displeased with the effect that drugs and surgery had on his patients. He found that when the bones and joints were in their proper place, the result was increased circulation and greater health. He traveled around teaching his techniques and eventually founded a school of osteopathic medicine in Missouri.

The second new healing practice that cropped up at this time was chiropractic.

THE FOUNDING OF CHIROPRACTIC

WHILE ANDREW SILL was looking into the relationship between joint manipulation and overall health another man, *David Daniel (D.D.) Palmer* was focusing on manipulation of one specific area -- the spine. Palmer was very interested in the causes of disease -- particularly

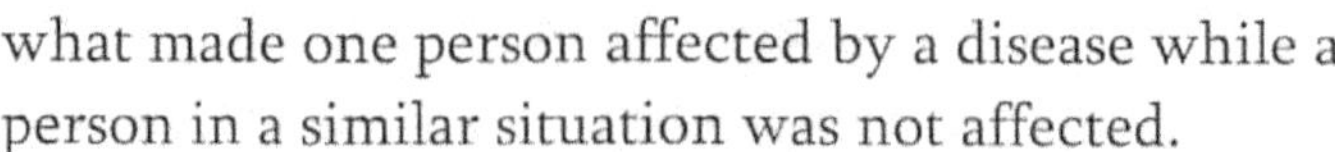

what made one person affected by a disease while a person in a similar situation was not affected.

His theory was that many illnesses and injuries could be attributed to a misalignment in the spine, which interfered with the nerve signals sent from the brain to the spinal cord to the rest of the body.

Palmer first tested his theory with an Iowa janitor named Harvey Lillard. Lillard, who had been deaf for 17 years, claimed he could hear until one day, when he was working, he bent over and felt something "go out" in his back. Palmer examined the man, found one of his vertebrae severely out of alignment, and using his hands pushed it back into place. Lillard's hearing was immediately restored.

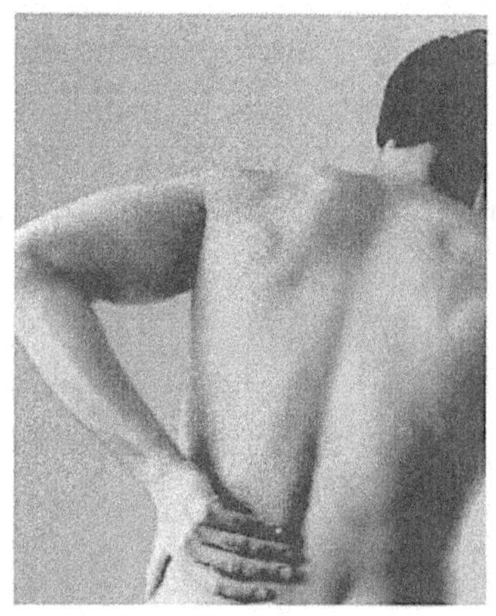

Palmer called his practice chiropractic, which comes from the Greek words cheri (hand) and praktikos (practice).

Palmer continued to work with patients with all different kinds of ailments, and many of them greatly improved with spinal manipulation. Over several years, as he saw more and more patients and honed his technique, what we know of today as chiropractic began

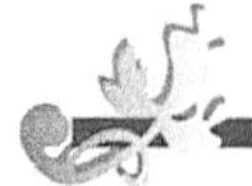

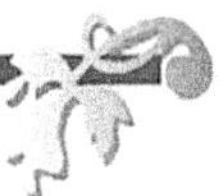

to take shape. The premises are few and easily understandable:

- ♣ Misalignments occur in the spine over time, either the result of trauma or misuse.

- ♣ These misalignments interfere with the flow of nerve impulses and energy -- communication, if you will -- between the brain, the spinal cord, and the body.

- ♣ When these nerve impulses are blocked, the body is no longer in its natural state and cannot function the way it was designed to. People with misalignments may experience limited motion, pain, or disease that may not appear to be related to the spine, but really is.

- ♣ By manually adjusting the spine, a chiropractor can bring the spine back into the correct alignment.

- ♣ When this is done the body once again is returned to its natural state. Communication is restored between the brain, nervous system, and body. Symptoms are alleviated and better health is enjoyed.

Since the early 20th century, the discipline of chiropractic has continued to grow and gain credibility. Palmer's son, B.J. Palmer, established chiropractic schools in several cities and states. There are now 18 accredited school in the United States and Canada, and all 50 states

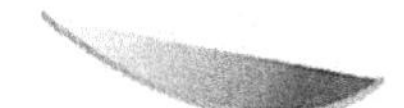

have a formal process, including licensing, that anyone wishing to practice chiropractic must follow. About 65,000 chiropractors practice in the U.S., while another 20,000 practice in other countries. Since the time of D. D. Palmer, chiropractic care has grown to be the second-largest health care system in the U.S., and the largest drug-free system in the world!

Sidebar: True Or False

OKAY, CHANCES ARE you picked up this book because you wanted to learn a little bit more about chiropractic care. Maybe you are giving chiropractic a try and want to understand it a little better. Or maybe it is something you are considering, but you are a little skeptical. One thing is for sure: there's lots of information out there about chiropractors and chiropractic care. Some of it is fact, and some of it is fiction! So, how do you know what to believe? Here are a few commonly held beliefs about chiropractors and chiropractic care. We'll tell you if they are True or False.

✍ Chiropractors are "quacks."

FALSE! Just like doctors, chiropractors are licensed medical professionals. Generally, students admitted to chiropractic school must have completed at least two years of undergraduate work, with an emphasis on

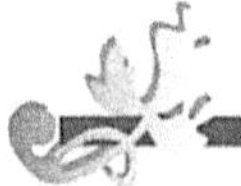

science. Chiropractic school takes four years and includes more than 2,880 hours of classroom instruction

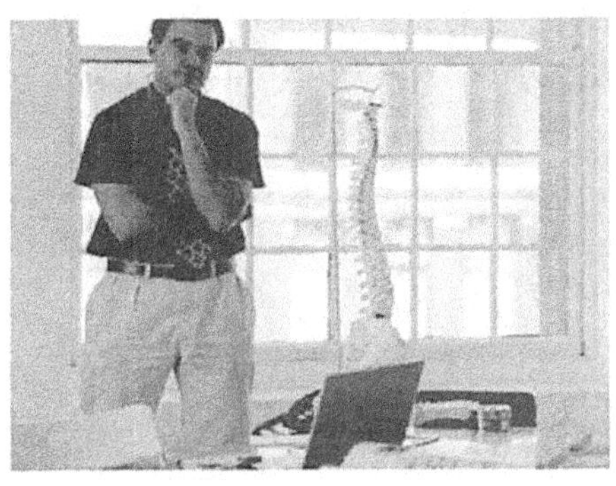

covering anatomy, physiology, chemistry, pathology, orthopedics, radiology, pediatrics, obstetrics, microbiology, neurology, diagnosis, geriatrics, and radiology. Like medical doctors, chiropractors see patients with a wide variety of illnesses and injuries. They must not only be able to manipulate the spine, they also need to be familiar with diagnosis and all facets of traditional medicine.

Once a chiropractor has graduated from school, he (or she) must do about 900 hours of work in a clinical setting, assisting other licensed chiropractors, before he can practice on his own. Once the student completes this apprenticeship he receives the doctor of chiropractic degree (D.C.). But wait! He can't hang out the shingle yet! First he must pass the state licensing exam, practical exam, and undergo an interview by the state. Once he passes all of the above, he can begin seeing patients. Doesn't sound easy, does it? As you can see, chiropractors have lots of training, knowledge, and experience before they open their doors to patients like you.

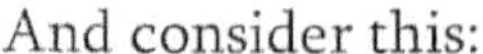

And consider this:

If chiropractors were "quacks" then federal and state programs like Medicare and Medicaid wouldn't cover chiropractic care, nor would the health insurance policies of more than 75 percent of the insurance carriers in the United States. Chiropractic is a recognized and well-respected aspect of our health care system!

✍ Chiropractic care is safe.

TRUE! There are no drugs that may have potentially dangerous side effects. No surgeries that may have complications. Chiropractic is natural. It is drug-free, surgery-free, and completely safe. The trained chiropractors working on your body have extensive knowledge of the spine and its alignment. They use only their hands to manipulate the spine and soft tissues. Chiropractic is completely safe!

✍ Chiropractic adjustments hurt.

FALSE! On the contrary, many chiropractic patients report an instantaneous relief of pain following their adjustments. If you think that chiropractors push, pull, and twist you, and that your back makes loud cracking noises during adjustments, think again! It only takes a minor misalignment for you to experience symptoms in your body, and therefore most chiropractic adjustments

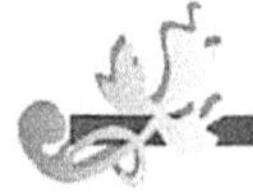

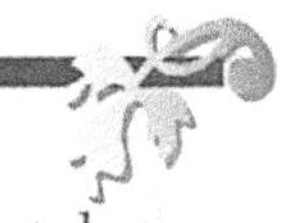

are quite subtle. It doesn't take much to put a vertebra back in its proper place, and most patients are still "waiting for something to happen" when they are told their adjustment is over!

> *You may experience minor muscle soreness for a day or two after adjustment as your muscles get accustomed to being used properly again, but all in all chiropractic does not hurt!*

✍ I don't need chiropractic care.

FALSE! Everyone needs chiropractic care. It is essential to optimal, on-going health and wellness. It's not possible to go through day-to-day life without your spine becoming misaligned. Whether it's because of a trauma, misuse, or overuse, our vertebrae are not always where they should be! Regular chiropractic care keeps things in order. You may not think you need it, but try it and see how much better you feel.

It's possible that those little things you've always accepted about yourself -- things you've decided to live with like stiffness, pain, or illness -- might actually resolve. Think your aches and pains are just a natural part of getting older? Well, think again! If you've never had chiropractic care, perhaps you can't even remember what your body feels like in its natural state. You'll be amazed at how much better you feel!

✍ Chiropractic care is for non-traditional
"New Age" people.

FALSE! Chiropractic is for everyone. It is for athletes,
parents, children, the elderly, pregnant women, people
who sit at their desks all day, and people who work
outside. Basically, chiropractic is for anyone who has a
spine! Twenty-five million people a year visit
chiropractors, and chances are some of them are your
neighbors, friends, and co-workers. So chiropractic is
certainly not just for those with New Age tendencies.

> *Rather, chiropractic is for anyone who wants to
> achieve better health in a natural, non-invasive,
> drug-free, proven way. And that probably means
> you!*

✍ You have to see your chiropractor
regularly to achieve any benefit.

TRUE and FALSE. If you are going to a chiropractor for
a specific reason -- let's use hip pain as a result of an
accident as an example -- then it's true that a certain
number of treatments will probably alleviate your hip
pain. So if the goal of visiting the chiropractor is only to
alleviate your hip pain, then no, you certainly do not
need to keep going for the rest of your life to reach that
goal.

But let's think back and remember the philosophy
of chiropractic care for a second here. Remember how

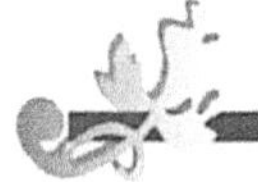

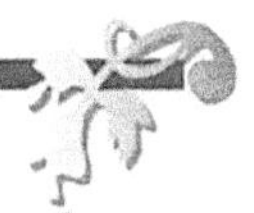

the philosophy of chiropractic is based on allowing the body to go back to its natural state, thereby ensuring better health and wellness? Well, if this philosophy is more in tune with your goals then yes, you'll want to schedule regular chiropractic care. In order to maintain your body's natural state, you'll have to take regular care of your spine.

How often should you go?

> *For preventive care, the recommended time is just one half-hour visit about every three months. Now that's a pretty small commitment when you consider the overall benefits, isn't it?*

⚕ Chiropractic cures diseases.

FALSE. *Chiropractic is focused on gaining health, not on curing specific diseases.* Chiropractic care is not designed to alleviate specific symptoms, like a pill. Instead, it is designed to promote a healthier body overall.

But when all is said and done, what is the result?

Well, if you have been reading carefully, you know that once the body reaches its natural state through spinal manipulation, pain and illnesses generally disappear. The body is healthier, and you feel as good as you can. So while the focus of chiropractic is not really to get rid of specific illnesses and injuries, it is an awfully nice side effect, don't you think? Curing disease is a great goal, but don't forget to make maintaining your health a goal in the first place. If you make maintaining your health a

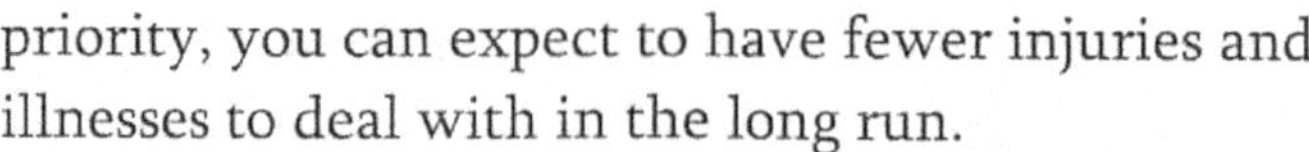

priority, you can expect to have fewer injuries and illnesses to deal with in the long run.

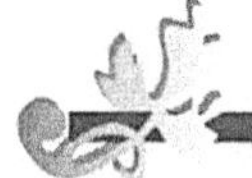 Insurance doesn't cover chiropractic care.

FALSE. As chiropractic gains credibility in the health insurance industry, more companies are including coverage for chiropractic care. Chances are, you can get coverage for chiropractic services through your regular health insurance plan. While some plans require you to be referred to a chiropractor by your primary care physician, others do not.

> *To find out whether your insurance policy covers chiropractic care, check your policy or contact the company's customer service department.*

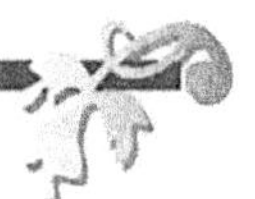

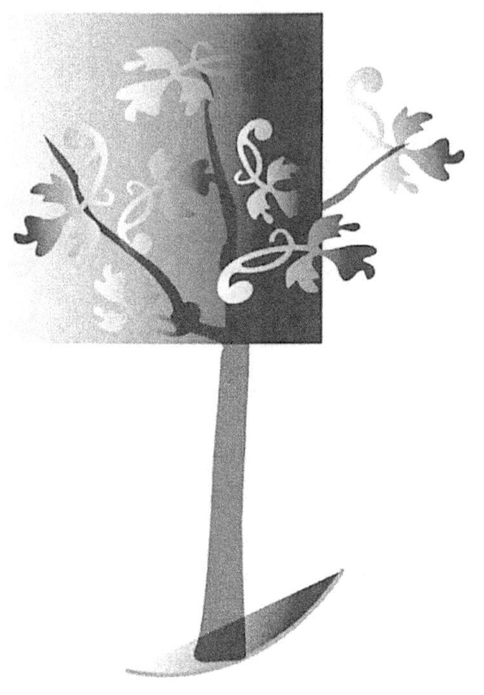

MOST PEOPLE THINK that chiropractors concentrate on the back and spine. Guess again. Chiropractors work primarily on the nervous system. *The body's nervous system -- comprising the brain, spinal cord, and nerves -- controls everything that goes on in the body.* It not only sends communication throughout the body, it connects the body to the brain.

CHAPTER
3

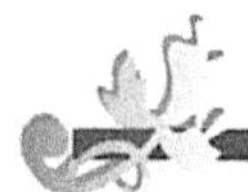

Chapter 3: How Chiropractic Works

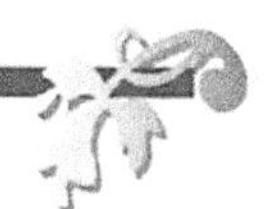

And what connects the brain to the rest of the body?

The spinal cord! If the spinal cord is healthy and aligned, then communication flows well throughout the body and allows it to enjoy good health. But sometimes there are problems with the spinal cord, specifically the vertebrae, which blocks communication.

What are vertebrae?

Vertebrae are the joints of the bones in the spine that wrap around the spinal cord. Their job is to protect the spinal cord. But everyday wear and tear, and sometimes misuse or an accident, can cause them to misalign, which prevents the spinal cord from functioning the way it should. The interferences are called subluxations. The goal of chiropractic is to remove these subluxations in order to restore the connections in our bodies, and help our whole bodies function as they should when they are in their natural state.

A LITTLE BIT ABOUT PAIN

WHAT'S THE POINT OF PAIN, anyway? Well, just like the engine light flashes in your car before it completely malfunctions, pain lets you know that something is not right with your body. When your engine light flashes you pull over and get it fixed, right? Similarly, pain lets us know that it's time to take action now, before further damage or injury occurs. No matter who you are, at some point in your life you'll experience pain. As a matter of fact, pain is one of the most prevalent health care problems in the United States today. It affects people from all over the country, from all walks of life, of all ages.

Pain is transmitted through the cells of the nervous system. It works this way: on one end of the nerve cell are little tendrils called dendrites. On the other side of the cell is a cord-like structure called an axon. Nerve cells are linked by these dendrites and axons, and nerve cell information is transmitted in the form of electrochemical impulses and neurotransmitters.

Nerves live just about everywhere in your body! They are in your arms, legs, toes, fingers, face, teeth, heart, liver, lungs, and intestines. They are in your eyes, stomach, tongue, nose, and skin. Some nerves are designed to provide sensory information like temperature, pressure, or pain, while others are designed to provide information on our physical movement. These nerve cells, which are interconnected, lead to the spinal cord, and then to the brain.

So how does pain happen?

In a nutshell, when nerve cells are irritated pain will happen. The pain message travels from the nerve cells to the spinal cord, and then to the brain, where we become aware of it.

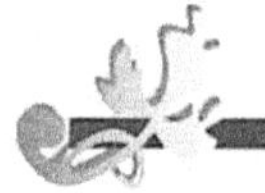

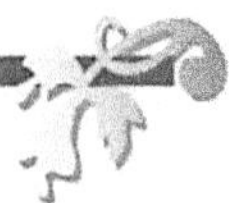

Let's break this down with an example you can understand.

Let's say you are playing tennis. You are hustling to get a short ball when you fall and twist your ankle. As soon as that ankle rolls over, nerve cells in the muscles and tendons send impulses through their axons. Chemicals called neurotransmitters are released. The neurotransmitters relay the message from the axon of one cell to the dendrites of another. The dendrites send the message to another axon, and so on and so on, the communication continues. The message eventually reaches the dorsal horn of the spinal cord, which is responsible for receiving information from the nerves. The information then goes to the thalamus, which is responsible for receiving sensory data and sending it to the cortex. Once the message gets to the thalamus, you'll know you are in pain! The brain will then send a message to the body telling it how to react; the message will go back through the spinal cord and through the nerves to the area that was injured. In the case of our tennis player's sprained ankle, the area will swell, turn colors, become tender to the touch and not allow pressure. And believe it or not, this will protect the ankle from being injured any more than it already is. How amazing is that?

Okay, so now that we've given pain a pretty positive spin, does this mean that you shouldn't try to relieve it? Absolutely not! Pain can have a widespread effect on our entire system. It doesn't just affect the area that was injured, but can also affect our organs, other bones and muscles, and even our mental processes. Chronic pain, or pain that occurs over a long period of time, is of particular concern, because after a period of time it takes fewer stimuli to provoke the same response.

Another issue is that while pain signals the body that something is wrong, it is not always accurate. Consider this: what is more dangerous, a broken bone or high blood pressure? High blood pressure, obviously. But what causes more pain? The broken bone.

> *The point is you can't really judge your overall health by the amount of pain -- or lack of pain, for that matter -- you are feeling. It's important to take care of yourself and promote good health well before the signals of pain start telling you something is wrong.*

CHIROPRACTIC AND PAIN

YOU NOW UNDERSTAND how the pain response works. You also understand that chiropractic's main focus is to make sure the nervous system is functioning to the best of its ability. If you put two and two together, you can see why chiropractic care is very effective at

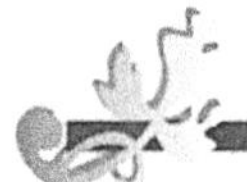

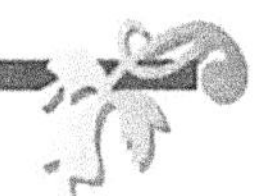

treating pain. It's easy to see why most people who visit chiropractors do so in order to alleviate or diminish pain.

Remember what we discovered about how conventional medicine treats pain? Most patients are offered drugs or surgery to combat pain, but drugs stop pain receptors from doing their jobs, and surgery can be dangerous, ineffective, or can cause even worse problems in the end.

So what's the answer? How do we combat pain?

The first step is to stop thinking that your goal is to alleviate pain. Instead, think of your goal as restoring function. When normal functioning is restored to the bones, tissues, and muscles, pain disappears. And that's a much better side effect than those of common anti-inflammatories, don't you think?

Why all this distinction between treating pain versus restoring function?

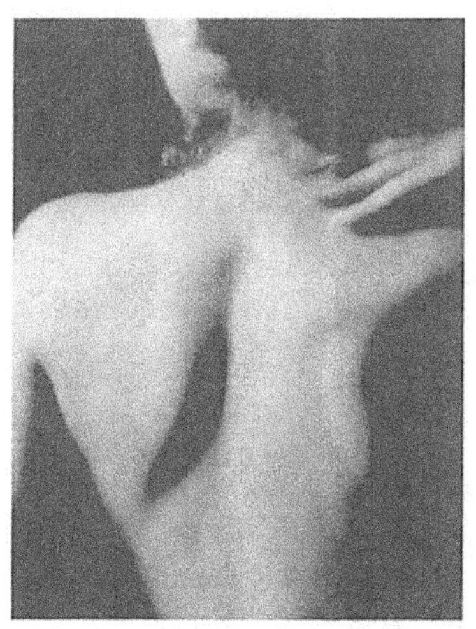

If pain is the patient's problem, and the chiropractor gets rid of it, then he's done his job, right? Not really. Let's say you have been in a car accident, and have hurt your lower back. You know you've hurt it because you feel pain. So you go and get some treatment. The treatment could include analgesics, ice, massage, or any other modality. The pain disappears, you stop treatment, and all is well. Right? Wrong! The accident caused loss of function in a particular area. The pain may have gone away, but your treatment plan did not focus on restoring full function. And if you don't have full function, you are not experiencing your best health.

Chiropractors know this, and that is why many of them prescribe a course of treatment regardless of whether the pain has gone away or not. A good chiropractor isn't just interested in taking away your pain, he or she is interested in correcting the reason why the pain occurred in the first place. If you can do that without drugs or surgery, then why wouldn't you?

COMMUNICATION AND THE SPINE

TO GET AN IDEA of the role the spine plays in communication throughout the body, think of those who have suffered severe spinal cord injuries. A paraplegic can't move his or her legs, but the legs were not the part of the body involved in the trauma. Instead, the problems are due to a spinal cord injury. There isn't really anything wrong with the legs themselves, they just aren't receiving communication from the brain and central nervous system. Which means they can no longer function.

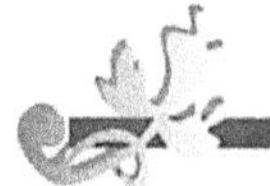

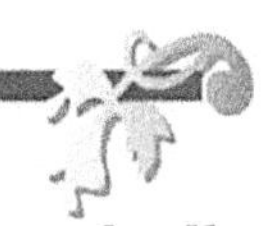

We experience lesser injuries to our spinal cords all the time, and these result in lesser problems, but problems just the same. Babies learning to walk fall down, kids get hurt roughhousing, athletes experience trauma or overuse, adults get in accidents or just get out of bed the wrong way. All of these things can cause misalignment.

The soft connective tissue around the spine can be damaged, and this can also cause problems. When these tissues are damaged, the vertebrae fall out of their correct alignment. Whether the impingement occurs with the bones of the spine or the connective tissue, it can interfere with the nerves. And when the nerves are interfered, with what happens? Well, if you've been reading carefully and paying attention, you know the answer is loss of function!

> *When the spine is put back into alignment, communication is restored and so is optimal body function. When the body is functioning the way it should it heals itself...and that is what chiropractic allows it to do.*

SUBLUXATIONS

WE'VE USED THIS WORD a few times in this text, and now it's time to properly define it.

> *Chiropractors define a subluxation as anything within the area of the spine that breaks the cycle of nerve communication between the brain and the body.*

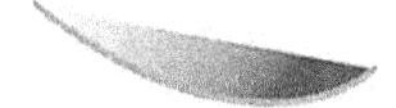

A subluxation results from trauma -- either an accident of some sort or continued misuse. Whether or not the alignment of the vertebrae shifts, there is almost always a loss in range of motion. You might experience stiffness, soreness, or lack of flexibility in your back and neck. You might have some pain, or you might not. Regardless, your body will be affected in some way!

But subluxations are complex, and the problems they cause are a little bit more widespread. When the vertebrae are out of alignment, the ligaments, tendons, cartilage, and muscles -- what we call connective tissue -- is also affected. Damage to the connective tissues, mostly in the forms of very, very small rips or tears, usually is painful and does result in inflammation.

What happens when this connective tissue swells?

All kinds of nasty things! If the damage is not treated the connective tissue between the vertebrae can wear away, resulting in a herniated or ruptured disk. When a disk is ruptured or herniated the vertebrae press on the spinal column. Ouch! Inflamed connective tissue also affects the bone it surrounds. Swollen, painful connective tissue doesn't allow you to move the misaligned bone the way you should. This means you move that part of the body in a way it isn't designed to move, causing even further damage.

Now that you understand how subluxations wreak local havoc, you are probably wondering how they interfere with the nervous system.

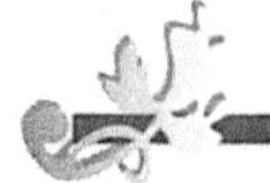

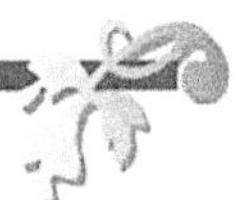

✅ They affect the flow of cerebrospinal fluid throughout the central nervous system.

Cerebrospinal fluid flows around the brain and spinal canal and provides nutrition and protection to both the spine and the nerves. A misalignment can cause the fluid not to flow properly, and this can prevent communication from flowing properly as well. The function of the nerves that attach to the cord can be affected as well.

Remember a few pages ago we discussed how pain is transmitted through the body? How it goes from nerve cell to nerve cell, along the spinal cord, to the brain, which decides how to handle the trauma (usually with pain and swelling) and then back again? Well, subluxations interfere with this loop. Because unless the cause of the trauma is corrected, the affected area continues to send out signals. The body will be overwhelmed by what it has to do -- it will not be able to handle all the healing it thinks it is supposed to be doing. The injury will either not heal, or it will get worse.

✅ The nerves going to the spinal cord and brain are affected. As the nerves continue to send out distress signals in the form of neurotransmitters, these neurotransmitters clog other nerve pathways in the spinal cord and brain. This affects communication throughout the body. And the results of this can show up anywhere in the body -- your arms, stomach, lungs, feet. Just about

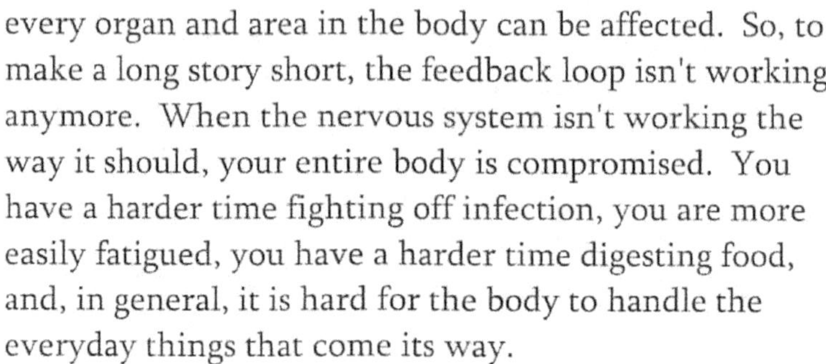

every organ and area in the body can be affected. So, to
make a long story short, the feedback loop isn't working
anymore. When the nervous system isn't working the
way it should, your entire body is compromised. You
have a harder time fighting off infection, you are more
easily fatigued, you have a harder time digesting food,
and, in general, it is hard for the body to handle the
everyday things that come its way.

Subluxations occur all the time, and most of the
time we're not even aware of them. And most of us
have them. They are unavoidable! Studies show that
95 percent of 45-year-olds have subluxations, while 80
percent of 20-year-olds do. And how many of us are
receiving regular chiropractic care? About 10 percent.
This means the other 90 percent of the population are
walking around with the communication between
their brains and central nervous system compromised.
This means that 90 percent of us are not enjoying the
best health we can.

So, if most of us are ignoring our subluxations,
what does this mean?

Subluxations eventually cause degeneration in the
muscles, bones, and nerves. Many people think that
aging brings on health issues like diminished mobility
and flexibility, waning vitality, and increased discomfort.
And in a way, this is true. The older you get and the
more you ignore your subluxations, the more you'll be

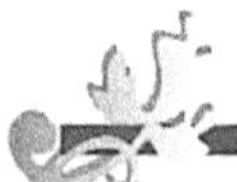

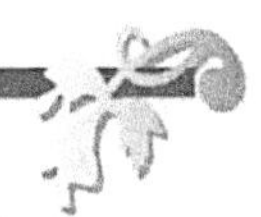

subject to diseases like arthritis, bone spurs, muscle weakness, and overall diminished health.

> *Remember, subluxations wreak havoc in all areas and organs of the body. However, if you receive regular chiropractic care, chances are you'll avoid these things. You'll feel and act much younger than people your age. Don't deny your subluxations, and chances are you'll experience great health! Remember, chiropractic treats nerves, not bones. Those nerves connect your entire system together. Take care of them!*

CHIROPRACTIC ADJUSTMENT: HOW IT WORKS

SO, HOW SHOULD YOU DEAL with the cycle of inflammation and injury that occurs with a subluxation?

As you remember -- taking anti-inflammatories is treating the symptom, not the underlying cause.

In chiropractic care, the cause of the problem is treated, not the symptoms. Chiropractors go right to the root of the problem -- the subluxations.

Think back to the philosophy of chiropractic, which states that the body is completely capable of healing itself. But sometimes it needs a little help due to interferences.

What causes these interferences? Misalignment of the spine, or subluxations.

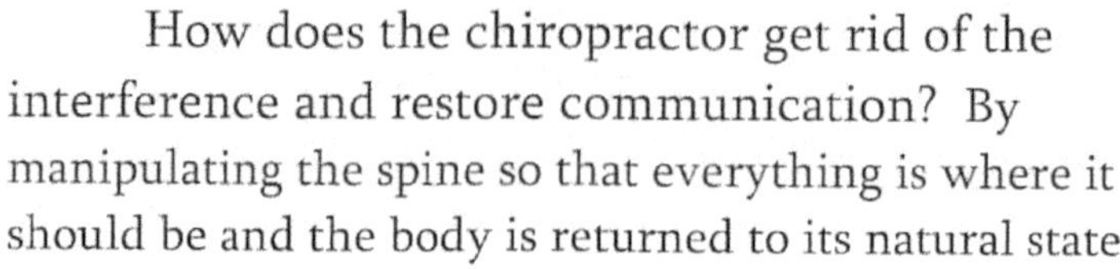

How does the chiropractor get rid of the interference and restore communication? By manipulating the spine so that everything is where it should be and the body is returned to its natural state.

Once everything is back in order, the body can begin to heal itself. In a typical chiropractic adjustment, the spine is aligned. When the spine is aligned, the connective tissue returns to normal. The adjustment also moves the bone through a range of motion, and this motion helps the neurotransmitters, which were in high alert before, go back down to normal levels. Once everything is back to normal the nervous system will once again be able to smoothly transmit messages between the brain and body. And you'll feel so much better!

Before you know it, the body is ready to start healing itself. You need to be a little patient at first. Don't expect results that same day! You might feel a slight bit of relief, or you might even feel a little muscle soreness the next day. That's completely normal. It takes a little while for the body to get back to optimal health, and sometimes, after using your body incorrectly for a period of time, your muscles will let you know you are using it correctly!

Notice how when we discuss chiropractic we use words like *"manipulate"* when speaking about the spine and subluxations. This is actually a very appropriately used word.

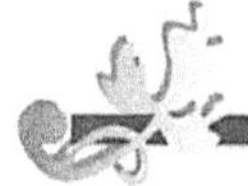

When a spine is manipulated -- when it is adjusted -- bones are not moved from out of place back into place. A vertebra isn't fixed -- there really isn't one place it should be. Instead, it has a normal range of motion. A subluxation causes this range of motion to be impeded -- either the vertebra is moving in an abnormal way, or it is locked outside of its normal range.

The chiropractor wants to unlock the joint from its locked position or incorrect way of moving, and he does this by pushing the joint beyond its lock, to the limit of its passive range of motion. A good analogy here is when you stretch. To get really limber and flexible you'll stretch as far as you can, and then you'll go a little farther. In a similar way, a chiropractic adjustment helps the joints remember their normal range of motion.

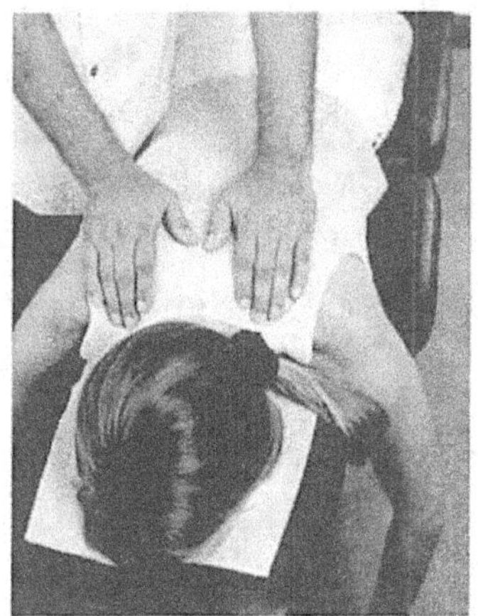

Let's talk a little bit about the passive range of motion versus the active range of motion.

The active range of motion is the amount you can move a joint on its own. Try this. Hold your hand straight up with the fingers pointing at the ceiling, and lay your wrist back. Now take your other hand and press down on the fingers of the hand you are moving.

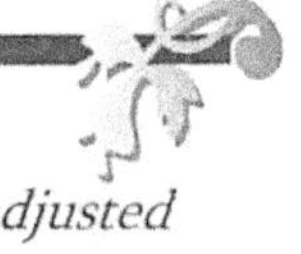

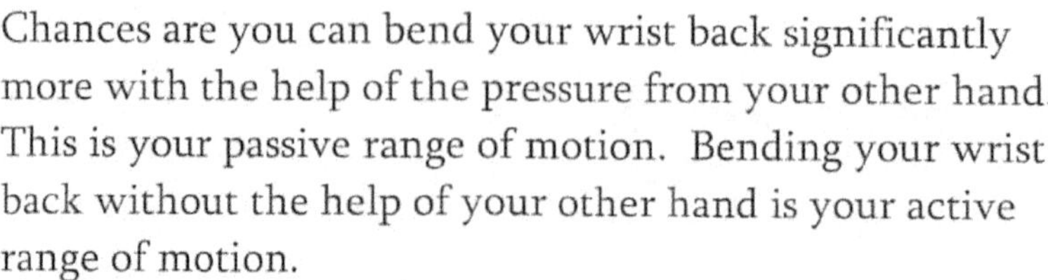

Chances are you can bend your wrist back significantly more with the help of the pressure from your other hand. This is your passive range of motion. Bending your wrist back without the help of your other hand is your active range of motion.

With a subluxation, your vertebra is locked at somewhere less than its active range of motion. So it can't even move on its own where it should. This limited range of motion results in abnormal motion, pain, the inflammation of the connective tissue, and all the effects of that we talked about earlier.

> *Chiropractic does what no medicine could ever do -- it treats the cause by restoring the normal range of motion -- first to the active range of motion, and then to the full passive range.*

We've talked a little bit about the philosophy of chiropractic, and you now probably have a good idea of how it works. Hopefully, you are now considering chiropractic care as one of your own health care choices. In the next section we'll give you an overview of certain conditions and how chiropractic is good for them. Just like in traditional medicine there are specialties and subspecialties in chiropractic care, and this section should help you choose a chiropractor that will suit your particular needs. We'll also explore several different populations -- people suffering injuries or illnesses, seniors, athletes, children, and pregnant women -- and show you how chiropractic care can benefit them.

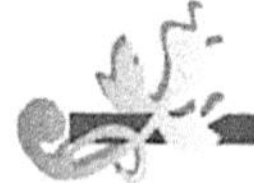

Chapter 3: How Chiropractic Works

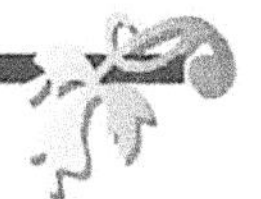

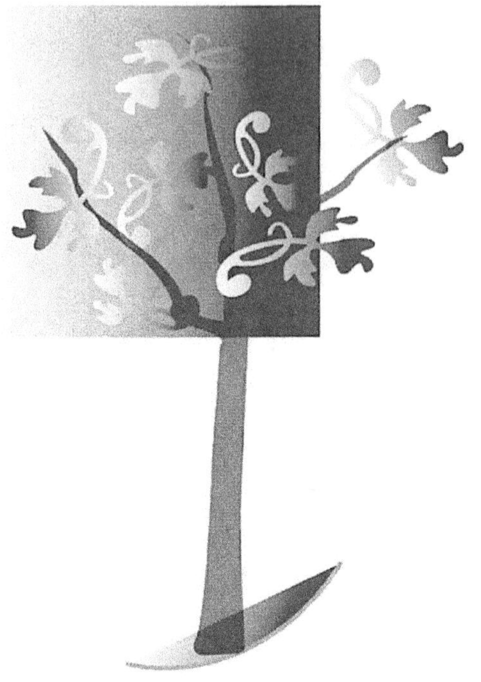

Who Needs Chiropractic?

EVERYONE! As stated before, everyday wear and tear causes subluxuations. And subluxations prevent you from enjoying your best possible health. So regular chiropractic care -- and by regular we mean about once every three months -- should keep you at your best.

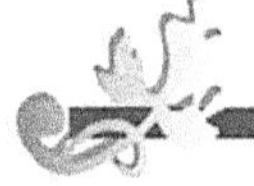

Think of it like going to a dentist. You go to the dentist twice a year whether or not you are having problems with your teeth, right? That's because maintenance is important. Well, the same principle applies to your spine. Maintenance is important.

It's important to note that while chiropractic should be an important part of your overall health plan, so should conventional medicine.

> *The best possible scenario is to have a team of doctors on your side -- both conventional and alternative. Your medical doctor should be accepting of and willing to work with your chiropractor, and vice versa. If you find that your current doctor has difficulty accepting alternative types of medicine, you might want to find someone else who has ideas about health care similar to yours.*

As we've mentioned several times before, the philosophy of chiropractic is not to treat symptoms. But once the body is operating as it should, patients often report not only an alleviation of symptoms, but also an improvement in conditions they might have. In fact, may people who seek chiropractic care do so because of their symptoms.

Scientific research has shown that chiropractic can help heal certain symptoms, conditions, and diseases. But how is chiropractic scientific research done?

There are two different kinds of scientific chiropractic research.

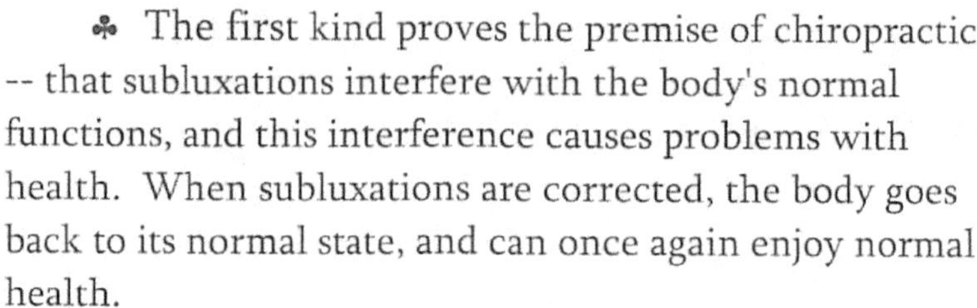

♣ The first kind proves the premise of chiropractic -- that subluxations interfere with the body's normal functions, and this interference causes problems with health. When subluxations are corrected, the body goes back to its normal state, and can once again enjoy normal health.

♣ The second kind of research looks at the effects of chiropractic care on specific conditions and diseases. Case studies make up the majority of this research. The results of chiropractic care on the conditions listed below are the result of many years of case studies and other types of research.

> Before you read the next section, it is important to note that while chiropractic can return the body to its optimal state, there are a number of different reasons why a disease or a condition might occur. Chiropractic can fix subluxations and help the body fight to heal itself, and sometimes this is all that is needed for a person to enjoy their best possible health. In other cases, chiropractic should be used in conjunction with traditional medicine, as part of an overall treatment plan. It is also important to note that there are some diseases and conditions that are unaffected by subluxations.

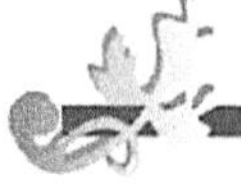

Chapter 4: Who Needs Chiropractic?

The following conditions are listed only as a guideline. *Please see your doctor for a diagnosis and treatment plan for your condition.*

CONDITIONS YOU MAY HAVE THOUGHT OF…

Back pain/sciatica.

CAUSE: Overuse, misuse, trauma, and everyday wear and tear.

> *This results in subluxations, muscle spasms, abnormal joint mechanics, and inflammation. How chiropractic helps: By getting rid of the subluxations, the muscles spasms, abnormal joint mechanics, and inflammation disappear.*

SUPPORTING STUDIES: A 1999 study compared chiropractic care, NSAIDs, and acupuncture.

> *Only those treated with chiropractic care showed significant improvement: 50 percent had less lower back pain, 46 percent had less upper back pain, and 33 percent had less neck pain.*

Cardiovascular health.

CAUSE: Studies show that cardiovascular health can be compromised when the upper thoracic vertebral joints are misaligned. This can cause problems with the sympathetic nerves that run to the heart and regulate

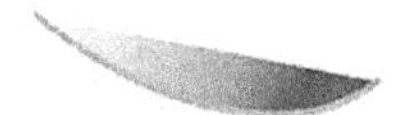

things like heartbeat rhythm.

How chiropractic can help: Aligning the spine restores function to the nerves.

SUPPORTING STUDIES:

A 1992 study showed that cholesterol levels were lowered for those who experienced regular chiropractic care.

Disk herniation and protrusion.

CAUSE: Continual soft tissue damage as a result of subluxations, trauma, or misuse.

How chiropractic care can help: Regular chiropractic care can maintain the back and spine

and prevent the degeneration from happening in the first place.

SUPPORTING STUDIES:

A 1996 study showed that 63 percent of participants had a reduction in herniation after receiving regular chiropractic care. Chiropractic shows a high degree of patient satisfaction as well.

Headache/migraine.

CAUSE: Many causes, ranging from subluxations to brain tumors.

How chiropractic care can help: For headaches caused by subluxations, usually in the neck, getting rid of the subluxations can result in relief in just a few visits.

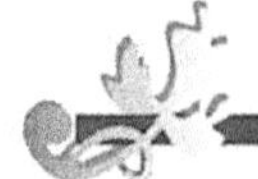

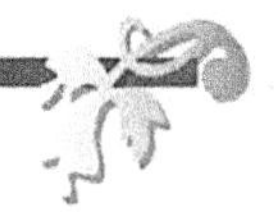

SUPPORTING STUDIES:

A 1994 study showed that 26 patients with headaches because of upper cervical joint dysfunction experienced fewer headaches with less severity when treated with chiropractic.

Knee problems.

CAUSE: Accident or issues with joint mechanics.

How chiropractic can help: When joint mechanics are involved, chiropractic care can correct issues of the spine that may be contributing.

Musculoskeletal conditions.

CAUSE: Trauma, injury, misuse, poor joint mechanics. How chiropractic can help: Almost any issue related to bones, muscles, and soft tissue can be resolved or improved using chiropractic care. A subluxation is often either the cause of the problem, or in the case of a trauma, the subluxation happened imultaneously.

Sinus problems.

CAUSE: Several causes, including cervical subluxations. How chiropractic can help: Adjustments of the spine and removing the cervical subluxations can help those with chronic sinus problems, as well as those with ear and tonsil issues.

☙ Torticollis.

CAUSE: The neck is twisted to one side. (This condition is usually seen at birth and is congenital.)

How chiropractic can help: Spinal adjustment, cranial work, and soft-tissue therapy have been shown to be effective alternatives to surgery.

☙ Trauma.

CAUSE: Accident or injury to a specific area of the body.

How chiropractic can help: Subluxations often occur at the same time as an injury or accident. Eliminating the subluxation speeds up the healing process.

☙ Whiplash.

CAUSE: Usually the result of trauma or an accident. Problems associated with whiplash include neck and back pain, headaches, and dizziness.

How chiropractic can help: Subluxations that don't show up on x-rays, and that occur at the time of the accident, are often the culprit. Correcting subluxations usually improves symptoms dramatically.

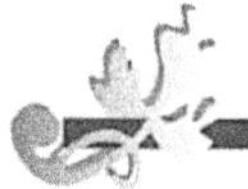

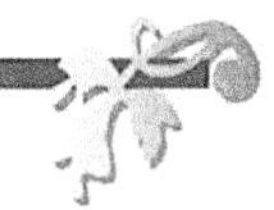

SIDEBAR: Chiropractic for Headache Sufferers

SINCE SO MANY OF US have battled with headaches to one degree or another at some point, it's well worth taking a little extra time here. Research shows that chiropractic care is highly effective for a variety of headaches, whether they are classified as migraine, tension, cluster, cervicogenic, or another type of headache.

Why is chiropractic helpful in treating headaches? Well, simply put, many headaches are the result of subluxations.

If your chiropractor's examination or x-rays indicate there is a misalignment in the neck region or cranial bones, chances are chiropractic care can help you

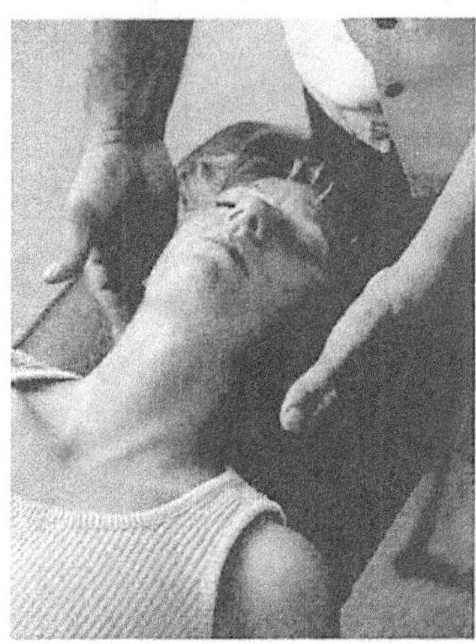

get rid of your pain. The nerves of the neck, when irritated, can lead to head pain that travels from the neck to the top of the skull and around the ears. Sometimes the pain can radiate to the face or eyes, and these types of headaches make clear thinking difficult. People who have suffered auto accidents or other types of traumatic injury often experience headache as a side effect, and this is often because vertebrae and/or soft tissue in the neck area have been injured.

It is important to note that headaches have many causes, and chiropractic care can't treat all of them. A chiropractor who does not see subluxations in the neck should not treat a patient for headaches; instead, the patient should seek traditional medical care to rule out other possible causes.

CONDITIONS YOU NEVER IMAGINED…

NOW GET READY for a really interesting list of conditions you probably never would've guessed chiropractic has been shown to successfully treat!

✍ Allergies.

CAUSE: Malfunction of the body's immune system response.

How chiropractic helps: By restoring health to the entire body, symptoms are reduced or eliminated. Supporting studies: 61.6 percent of children with various complaints, including allergies, were shown to improve in a 1988 study done at Western Chiropractic College.

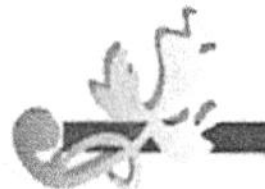

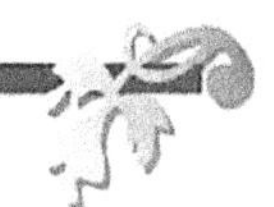

✍ Asthma.

CAUSE: Dilation of the bronchial tubes due to allergens; can also be induced by exercise, stress, and other situations.

SUPPORTING STUDIES:

> *Study done in 1997 showed that 90.1 percent of kids with asthma improved after two months of chiropractic care. A 1995 study showed that 95 percent of adults with asthma improved both peak flow rate and vital capacity after the third visit with their chiropractor.*

✍ ADHD.

CAUSE: Behavior and biochemical disorder that causes difficulty paying attention, lack of impulse control, hyperactivity, and other behavior issues.

How chiropractic helps: Parents seeking non-drug alternatives are turning to options like chiropractic.

SUPPORTING STUDIES: The effectiveness of chiropractic for treating this condition has been known for decades.

> *A 1980 study gave half the children participating a drug, the other half chiropractic care. Those in the chiropractic group had decreased hyperactivity and improved attentiveness, as well as improved gross and fine motor skills. Those who took the drug also experienced less hyperactivity and more attentiveness, but had to take an increased dosage*

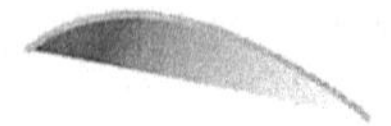

of drugs to keep the effect up. Fine and gross motor skills showed no improvement.

♋ Brain function.

CAUSE: Blood flow to the brain can possibly be impeded by subluxations causing problems such as memory loss vision issues, and emotional changes.

How chiropractic can help: Getting rid of subluxations causes optimal blood flow to the brain.

♋ Constipation.

CAUSE: Diet, and sometimes subluxations in specific areas of the spine.

How chiropractic can help: Removal of the subluxations helps the bowels function properly again.

♋ Diabetes.

CAUSE: Lack of proper insulin production.

How chiropractic can help: Diabetics sometimes lose feelings in their legs and feet due to circulation problems, which can lead to the loss of a limb. Chiropractic care can reduce this risk and also help the patient cut down on the amount of insulin taken. Supporting studies: A 1989 study showed diabetics who received regular chiropractic care were able to decrease their insulin intake. Another study done in 1989 and again in 1994 showed diabetic

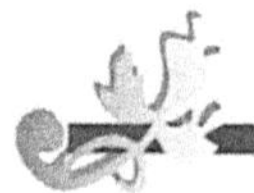

Chapter 4: Who Needs Chiropractic?

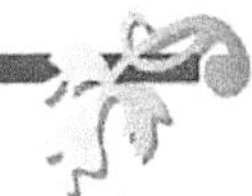

patients who experienced chiropractic care felt warmth
and a return of feeling in previously numb feet and legs.

✍ Ear infections.

CAUSE: Bacteria, fluid.

How chiropractic can help: By restoring balance in the
body, it heals itself. The body is better able to fight
infection without the use of antibiotics.

SUPPORTING STUDIES:

> *A 1997 study followed 332 children with ear
> infections, and showed that all the children showed
> improvement of the condition with only
> chiropractic care.*

✍ Epilepsy/seizures.

CAUSE: Electrical discharge from the nerve cells of the
cerebral cortex, resulting in rigidity and convulsions.
How chiropractic can help: By restoring a healthy
connection between the brain, body, and central nervous
system.

SUPPORTING STUDIES:

> *A 1992 study showed reductions in negative brain
> wave activity, and also a reduction in the frequency
> of seizures in children who had regular chiropractic
> care.*

Immune system dysfunction.

CAUSE: A number of reasons, including issues with the nervous system.

How chiropractic can help: By restoring communication between the brain, body, and nervous system.

SUPPORTING STUDIES:

A 1994 study of AIDS patients who received regular chiropractic care showed a 48 percent increase in immune response.

Infertility.

CAUSE: A variety of causes, including subluxations in the lower spine.

How chiropractic can help: By reducing subluxations in the lower spine, heightened fertility levels can occur.

Internal organ disease.

CAUSE: Many, including displacement of the spine, which can affect the nervous system, resulting in a wide variety of issues in the body, including issues with the organs.

How chiropractic can help: treating related parts of the spine can cut down on symptoms and sometimes even cure problems with internal organs.

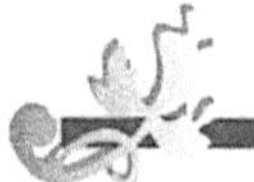

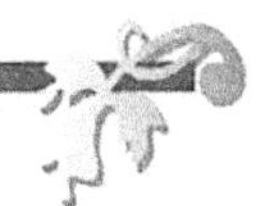

♋ Lung and respiratory problems.

CAUSE: A variety of different causes.

How chiropractic can help: The lungs are connected to the spine by nerves. Good spine alignment has a great effect on the respiratory system. It can increase both airflow and lung capacity, as well as help heal conditions related to the respiratory system more quickly.

♋ Pregnancy-related issues.

CAUSE: Weight gain, plus pressing of the fetus on the nerves and trunk, can cause back and spinal problems.

How chiropractic can help: Provides drug-free alternative to elimination of pain and overall health of mother.

SUPPORTING STUDIES:

> *A 1987 study by the American Medical Association showed that women in their third trimester of pregnancy who had chiropractic care carried their babies to term and delivered them in greater comfort.*

♋ PMS.

CAUSE: Hormonal shifts cause back pain, bloating, mood swings, breast sensitivity, depression, and impaired cognitive ability.

How chiropractic can help: Women with PMS might have a spinal dysfunction that causes these problems. Manipulating the spine can help to alleviate symptoms.

❧ Stuttering.

CAUSE: Physical, behavioral, and emotional causes, as well as an obstruction in communication between the brain, nerves, and muscles in the mouth.

How chiropractic can help: By aligning the spine the communication between the brain, nerves, and body is improved.

❧ TMJ.

CAUSE: the joint that connects the jawbone to the temporal bone is not functioning properly and/or is causing pain.

How chiropractic can help: By eliminating any subluxations, either cranial or cervical, that may be contributing to the condition.

❧ Ulcers.

CAUSE: Many different causes, including displacement of the spine that causes issues with internal organs.

How chiropractic can help: Manipulation of the spine returns full function to organs; promotes faster healing.

SUPPORTING STUDY:

> *A 1993 study showed that patients with duodenal ulcers who also had chiropractic care had faster healing times and less pain than those who didn't receive chiropractic care.*

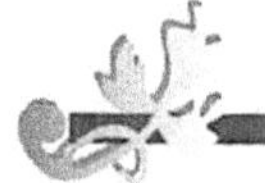

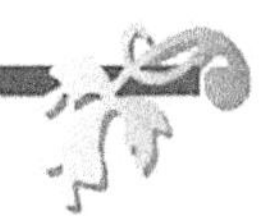

ॐ Vision problems.

CAUSE: Many, including impingement on the nerves that run to the eyes.

How chiropractic care can help: Chiropractic treatments on the upper cervical area can improve eyesight.

SUPPORTING STUDIES:

> *A 1996 study showed that blurred vision, contraction of the visual field, spots before the eyes, eye muscle dysfunction, and dry eyes were greatly improved by chiropractic care.*

CHIROPRACTIC FOR OLD AND YOUNG ALIKE!

WE'VE ALREADY SEEN how chiropractic works, and how it can ease symptoms and conditions. But chiropractic is great for healthy people in certain populations as well. Chances are you fit into one of the following categories, or know someone who does!

CHIROPRACTIC FOR SENIORS

THINK OF THE MANY THINGS we associate with aging -- frailty, increased aches and pains, decreased cognitive ability, less energy, lowered resistance to disease, and decreased mobility. Are these the inevitable realities of

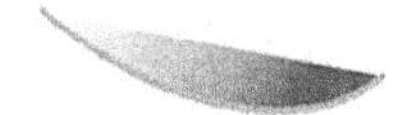

getting older? Should we just accept them and learn to deal with them? Absolutely not! Chances are you know a senior or two who has somehow managed to defy aging as we know it.

What's the difference between these types of seniors and those who have a laundry list of age-related issues?

Most likely, the seniors in the former category have taken good care of their bodies throughout the years. They have exercised, eaten well, and gotten plenty 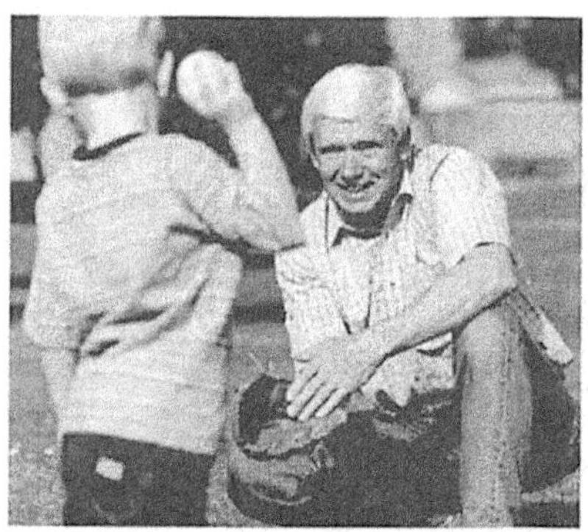 of sleep. They have treated their bodies well and have asked their bodies to function at the highest possible level. And a great way to keep your body functioning at the highest possible level is to get regular chiropractic care. As we discussed earlier, regular chiropractic care fixes subluxations before they can get around to doing a lot of damage. It's a great way to stay in optimal health!

Remember that chiropractic treats the nerves, joints, bones, and spine and helps them reach their best levels of function. Seniors who choose chiropractic care because of pain often get the added rewards of better overall health and vitality.

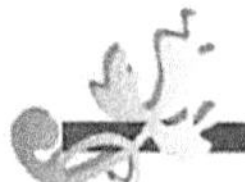

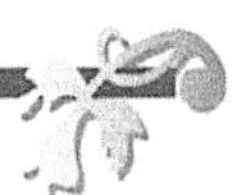

Regardless of how old we are chronologically, we are only as old as we feel! And how old we feel is often determined by how we have treated our bodies over the years. If you've treated your body well, chances are you'll experience less degeneration than someone whose body has been stressed over the years. And chiropractic care is one of the best ways to treat your body well.

Subluxations that go untreated will result in inflammation and deterioration of soft tissue, and that can lead to degeneration over time. With degeneration comes nerve interference, osteoarthritis, muscle weakness, and bone spurs.

These things may be minor in the beginning -- maybe even unnoticeable -- but over time, if left untreated, they will become more pronounced. And they'll speed up the aging process too, which none of us need!

Aches and pains, limited mobility, frailty, cognitive impairment -- these things are not necessarily just signs of aging, so don't accept them as such. A few minor adjustments can make all the difference in the world and improve the quality of living of many seniors. Most seniors need regular care to get the joints moving and repair the damage that has occurred over the years. Maintenance of the spine and nervous system can increase vitality and mobility, lessen pain, and improve nerve function. Seniors who are more mobile and experience less pain can also exercise more, which further increases health.

Seniors who have more than normal thinning of disks and bone spurs may have untreated subluxations. This degeneration, when untreated, can turn into osteoarthritis of the spine and neck. And many seniors seek chiropractic care when they get to this point.

A good way to avoid osteoarthritis in the first place is to get regular chiropractic care, which will help your body avoid the soft tissue inflammation that eventually causes it.

If you already have osteoarthritis, all is not lost! Chiropractic care can slow down the process, and sometimes even stop it. Once those pesky subluxations are eliminated and all is flowing well between the nerves, brain, and body, patients experience more energy and greater mobility and flexibility.

Can chiropractic "cure" degeneration?

Unfortunately, no. An impaired nerve that is no longer able to function or a disk that is thinned cannot be repaired by chiropractic, no matter how many treatments you have.

So what's the point if you have reached this stage?

Well, good chiropractic care will get you functioning at the highest level possible, and that is quite a benefit! Even a small amount of care will make a huge difference in how a senior feels on a day-to-day basis.

Those other conditions that seem to plague the elderly -- things like difficult breathing, constipation,

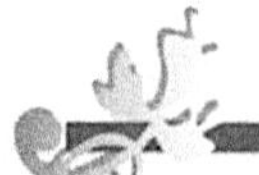

and digestion -- are also positively affected by chiropractic adjustments. Remember that chiropractic is a treatment of the nervous system, and all of the above conditions are impacted by nervous system function.

> *To this end, it is not uncommon for a senior to seek chiropractic care for pain, and get the extra added benefit of increased lung capacity! That's pretty exciting, don't you think? It will certainly cut down on the amount of medications the senior needs to take. Just think about saying goodbye to your laxatives, NSAIDs, sleeping pills, and energy boosters. How great would that be?*

CHIROPRACTIC FOR KIDS

ON THE OPPOSITE END of the spectrum, you might not know this but chiropractic is great for kids! It is a wonderful way to promote healthy living and deal with childhood illnesses and injuries without the use of drugs and surgery.

> *Chiropractic is perfectly safe for children; in fact, children are easy to adjust because their spines and bones are more malleable than those of adults.*

Kids take lots of falls and tumbles. They are active, and their active lifestyles result in more than a few bumps and bruises. Babies fall while learning to walk, toddlers learning to ride bikes take a few tumbles, and kids are pushed down and bumped into on the playground. The youthful bodies of children are meant

to take such abuse, and it's rare for these happenings to cause significant pain and injury. They can cause subluxations, however, and it is important for these to be resolved. A properly aligned spine helps a child develop healthily.

> *Regular chiropractic care can train a child's bones, joints, nerves, and muscles to function to the best of their ability. Kids don't need a lot of care -- healthy kids without specific pain or conditions should be seen about once every three months just to keep things in check.*

What if a child has an accident or injury?

Well, you should definitely see your child's pediatrician; in an emergency you should go straight to the hospital. But you should also see your chiropractor to check the child's spinal health. If your child sees a chiropractor regularly and is in no pain, it's fine to wait until the next scheduled visit. Kids with specific injuries might want to get in a little sooner. Kids who play sports should also see a chiropractor regularly. Like adult athletes, very active kids put more than the usual amount of stress on the body. To keep it functioning at its peak, chiropractic care is strongly recommended. The demand young athletes place on their bodies can cause damage to their bones, muscles, and joints; chiropractic care helps the body heal itself.

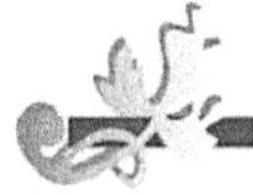

Chiropractic is also known to help such common childhood illnesses such as ear infections, tonsillitis, digestive problems, and allergies. How?

Well, there is a connection between the spine and the immune system, so it stands to reason that if the spine is in good health, then the immune system will be too. Subluxations cause communication issues between the nerves that run from the spinal cord to the organs and limbs. The tissues in these areas 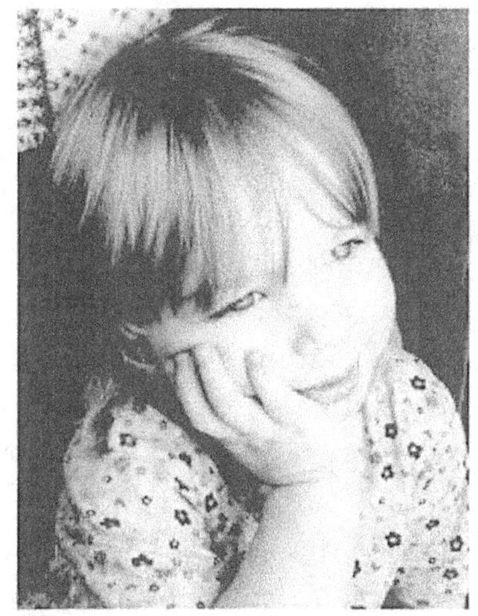 are eventually affected, and this is when we start to see some of the above conditions.

So chiropractic can be a great, drug-free way to keep your kids healthy. Aren't adjustments a more attractive alternative to rounds of antibiotics and all their side effects?

Make chiropractic a part of your family's health regimen. Let your kids enjoy its benefits. Showing your kids how the body can heal itself while also promoting optimal health is a wonderful gift indeed.

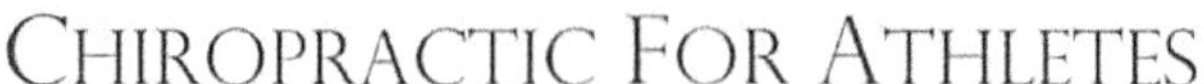

CHIROPRACTIC FOR ATHLETES

THERE'S PROBABLY NOT a healthier population than athletes. Think about it -- athletes exercise, eat right, and are concerned with their bodies and their performance. But athletes can really benefit from chiropractic care. Athletes are harder on their bodies than non-athletes. They push themselves to perform by logging lots of hourstraining, whether they are running, swimming, playing tennis, or lifting weights. The amount of time athletes put into their pursuits is really amazing! It seems very counter-productive then when all that hard work and effort result in injuries, both major and minor. Nothing can sideline an athlete faster or halt progress than an injury!

Injuries athletes generally face include cranial, spinal, and extremity contusions, strains, sprains, fractures, subluxations, dislocations, and soft tissue trauma.

Chiropractic care has become popular with athletes recently, mostly due to press regarding professional athletes' successful use of chiropractic as a health care system, as well as endorsement by Olympic athletes. And it is no wonder. *In addition to helping relieve and alleviate common symptoms athletes face such as inflammation and pain, chiropractic keeps the body in fighting shape. This means that athletes with injuries recover from them faster, as the body in its natural state helps to heal itself.*

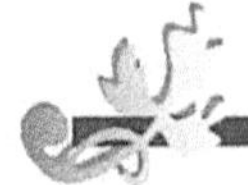

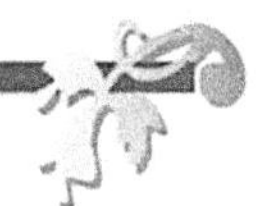

Athletes generally see chiropractors in conjunction with other health professionals such as physical therapists and sports medicine doctors.

As an example, let's take a tennis player with an injured and painful Achilles tendon. A sports medicine doctor might prescribe rest and anti-inflammatories, and might suggest a course of physical therapy. Physical therapy might include such modalities as ultrasound or iontophoresis to relieve pain and inflammation. Chiropractic care would round out the treatment nicely by removing subluxations that might be contributing to -- or preventing the full recovery of -- the injury.

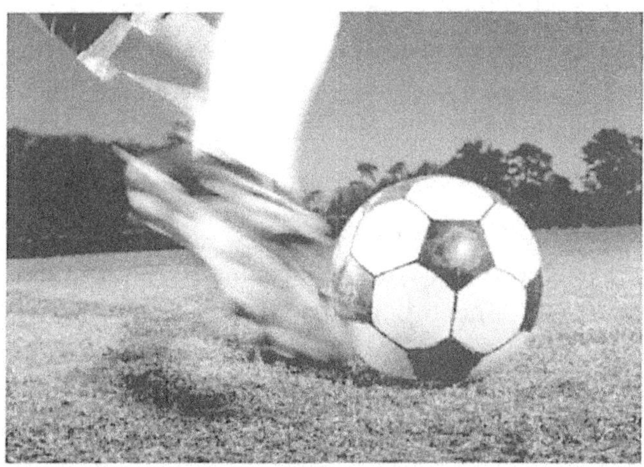

Since sports chiropractic has developed at a considerable pace, there are chiropractors who specialize in this field. These chiropractors are used to dealing with athletes, so they also keep abreast of the latest developments and advances in sports medicine. Athletes should not have too much difficulty finding a chiropractor who is experienced in treating sports-minded individuals.

CHIROPRACTIC FOR PREGNANT MOMS

THERE'S NOTHING LIKE carrying an extra 25 to 35 pounds to increase stress on the body and make you uncomfortable. That's why about half of all expectant moms develop lower back pain during their pregnancies.

Why is carrying a baby so uncomfortable?

Well, during pregnancy, mom's center of gravity shifts forward to the front of her pelvis and increases the stress on her joints. As the baby grows and mom's weight is projected even further forward, the curvature of the lower back is increased, placing extra stress on the spinal disks. To compensate, the normal curvature of the upper spine increases too. Ouch!

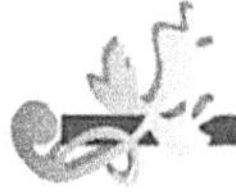

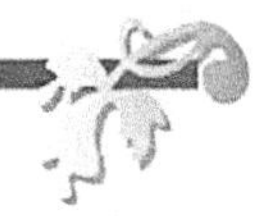

In a nutshell, that back pain is almost always the cause of subluxations. The subluxations, in turn, cause muscle spasms and stress on the spine and nerves. And what does that result in? Yes, you guessed it. Pain!

But never fear, your chiropractor can help! If you are trying to get pregnant, let your chiropractor know. He or she will be able to detect any imbalances in the pelvis or elsewhere in the body that could contribute to pregnancy discomfort or possible neuromusculoskeletal problems after childbirth.

Many pregnant women also find that chiropractic adjustments increase their level of comfort during pregnancy, especially when that discomfort is related to the lower back.

But are chiropractic adjustments safe during pregnancy?

Absolutely! Chiropractic care is becoming a lot more common during pregnancy. Lots of OBs give it a ringing endorsement. If yours doesn't, you might want to shop around for another doctor whose philosophy on

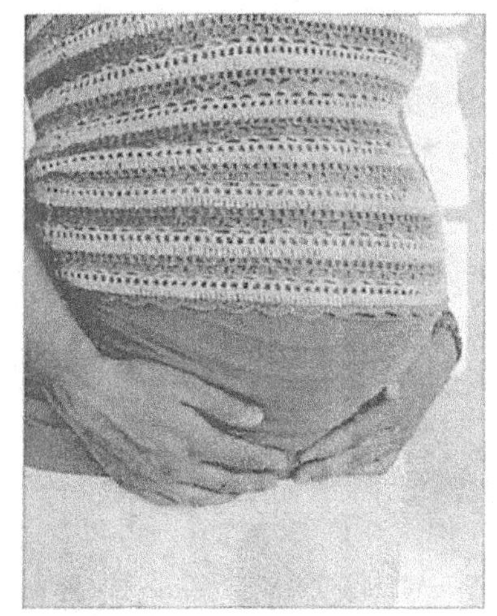

health care is more similar to yours. You probably won't

have to look too hard to find one who is open to the concept!

Chiropractic care is safe for both the mom and her baby, and is a great alternative to pain-killing drugs. Many doctors of chiropractic can also offer advice about exercise and nutrition which will increase your enjoyment of the pregnancy.

How about chiropractic following delivery?

Yes! During pregnancy, ligaments relax to allow for extra room in the pelvis. But in the eight weeks following labor and delivery, those ligaments that loosened begin to tighten up again. Joint problems brought on by pregnancy should be treated before the ligaments return to their pre-pregnancy state to prevent muscle tension, headaches, rib discomfort, and shoulder problems.

The American Chiropractic Association (ACA) also recommends the following practices for pregnant women:

♣ Exercise at least three times per week, and don't forget to stretch before each session. Safe exercises for pregnant women include those that do not require jerking or bouncing, like walking, swimming, and stationary cycling.

♣ Pay attention to ergonomics! Sleep on your side with a pillow between your knees to take pressure off your lower back. Lie on your left side, which will allow unobstructed blood flow and helps your

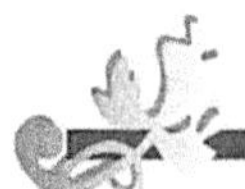

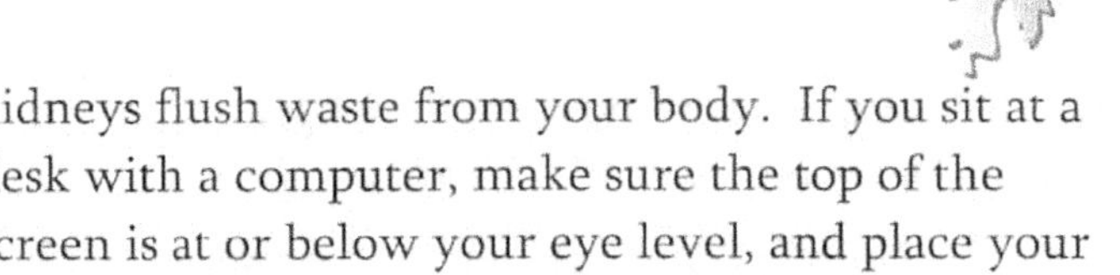

kidneys flush waste from your body. If you sit at a desk with a computer, make sure the top of the screen is at or below your eye level, and place your feet on a footrest to take pressure off your legs and feet. Take breaks to walk and stretch every 30 minutes or so.

- ♣ Instead of three large meals, eat four or five smaller meals to keep nausea and hunger at bay. Supplement your diet with 400 micrograms of folic acid per day.

Adding chiropractic care to her health care regimen is a great way for a woman to enjoy a healthy, pain-free pregnancy!

Chiropractic For Optimal Health

IT IS NO COINCIDENCE that most chiropractors are also well-versed in exercise, nutrition, and stress reduction, and offer this type of counseling to their patients. Since chiropractic is focused on treating causes, not symptoms, of disease, it just makes sense that doctors of chiropractic encourage their patients to lead healthy lifestyles.

Sure, subluxations are often caused by trauma or by everyday wear and tear. But they are also caused by lifestyle choices that impact our overall health -- choices

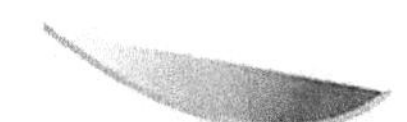

like smoking, eating the wrong foods, or sitting in front of the television instead of getting regular exercise.

Remember one of the main tenets of chiropractic -- health and well-being come from within and we have control -- and responsibility -- over our own health. We all have choices to make, and those choices will affect our overall health.

In the early 1900s, chiropractors used the term "survival values" to determine the impact our choices made on our health and life. The idea was simple: all of the choices we make either increase or decrease our chances of survival. And the same holds true today. Smoking decreases your chance of survival. Eating healthfully increases your chance for survival.
And how does chiropractic fit into all of this?

Well, chiropractic, as you know, returns your body to its natural state and allows it to heal itself.

So regular chiropractic care definitely increases your chance of survival. And your chiropractor wants you to eat well, get regular exercise, and manage your stress, because it is part of a healthy lifestyle, just like chiropractic. Healthy living and chiropractic go together. Sure, you can have one without the other, but you get the most out of both when you use them together!

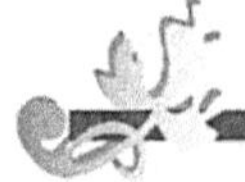

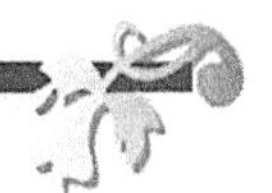

Different Kinds Of Chiropractors

ONCE YOU'VE DECIDED that chiropractic care is an avenue you want to take to promote better health, you'll have to take on the task of finding a chiropractor who fits your needs. With almost 50 different techniques used in chiropractic, that can be a daunting task.

CHAPTER
5

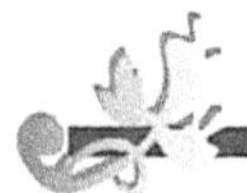

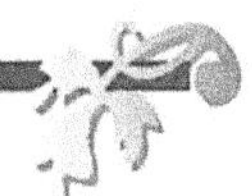

Add to that the fact that there are chiropractors who specialize in just about every population -- kids, seniors, athletes, people who have been injured or in accidents -- and the choice becomes even more difficult. What's more, chiropractors have different styles and philosophies.

But hold on. Take a deep breath and relax. Choosing a chiropractor doesn't have to be hard. As long as you know the kind of treatment you need, look for chiropractors who offer that treatment, then confirm your choice by asking a few pertinent questions, and you should have a good experience. Make an informed choice just like you would with any other health professional, and your needs will be met.

We mentioned earlier that within chiropractic there are just about 50 techniques that are used. Before you get too worried, you should know that you don't need to examine all 50. All chiropractic care falls within three main categories. If you familiarize yourself with these three categories, you'll be able to choose the type of care that is best for you. The three types of chiropractic are straight, mixing, and allopathic.

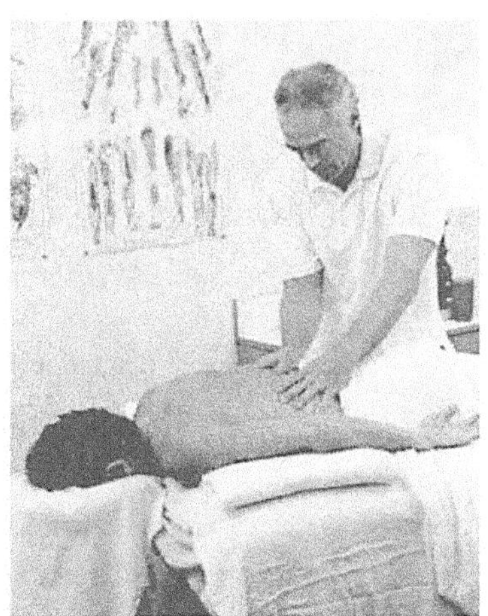

Straight Chiropractic Care

CHIROPRACTORS WHO PRACTICE straight chiropractic believe that the body has the ability to heal itself with little intervention.

> *Straight chiropractic is sometimes also called subluxation-based chiropractic, and its main premise is that subluxations cause poor health and prevent the body from healing itself. The goal of the subluxation-based chiropractor is to adjust the spine so that subluxations are eliminated. Straight chiropractors specialize in spinal manipulation, and while they believe that this spinal manipulation has a great effect on the entire body and its health, they usually offer their services in conjunction with traditional medicine, not instead of traditional medicine.*

Mixing Chiropractic Care

MIXING CHIROPRACTORS offer services in addition to spinal adjustments.

> *Treatment of subluxations is often still the main treatment of mixing chiropractics, but they also offer other modalities to support spinal adjustment. Some mixing chiropractors use alternative medicine, some use traditional medicine, and some use a combination of the two. If you go to a mixing chiropractor, chances are you'll receive treatment in addition to your adjustment.*

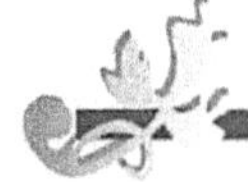

Chapter 5: Choosing A Chiropractor

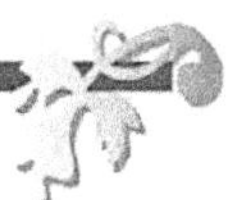

This treatment might consist of massage, homeopathy, or naturopathy. Sometimes services like nutritional counselling or emotional counselling will be available. Like straight chiropractic care, mixing chiropractic care strives to heal the body naturally. But it attempts to do so without the help of conventional medicine.

ALLOPATHIC CHIROPRACTIC

THIS TYPE OF CHIROPRACTIC is a smaller school than either straight or mixing. Allopathic chiropractors have something in common with traditional medical doctors, and that is that their goal is to treat symptoms.

> *Allopathic chiropractors are concerned with treating back pain, and not with eliminating subluxations. They do not focus on the potential underlying causes, but rather focus on relieving symptoms. Allopathic chiropractors usually treat patients for a short course -- usually six sessions or so -- and if things haven't improved refer them to a medical doctor for further treatment.*

So, what kind of chiropractor should you see?

- ♣ If you are interested in promoting overall health through spinal adjustments, you should see a straight chiropractor.

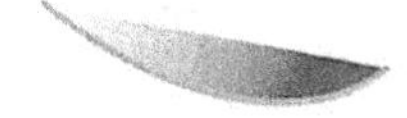

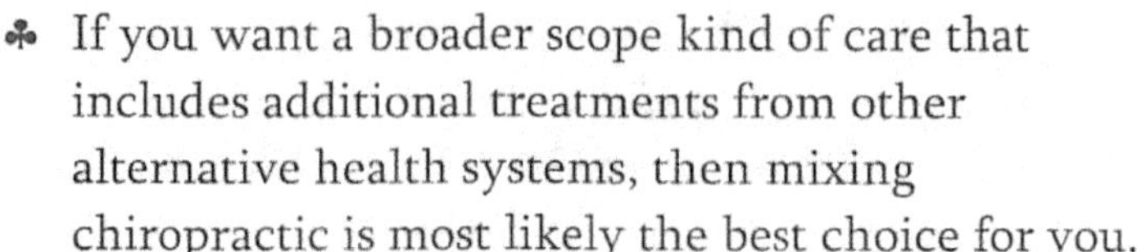

- ♣ If you want a broader scope kind of care that includes additional treatments from other alternative health systems, then mixing chiropractic is most likely the best choice for you.

- ♣ If you are most comfortable with traditional medicine and are looking for relief of specific symptoms, then allopathic chiropractic might be the ticket.

Once you've decided whether to go with a straight, mixing, or allopathic chiropractor, you'll need to narrow your choice down even more.

There are many, many different schools of chiropractic technique, and one of them is right for you. Two of your main concerns should be whether or not the chiropractor focuses on a specific area of the spine, and how much force her or she uses in adjustments.

DIFFERENT CHIROPRACTIC TECHNIQUES

DIFFERENT TECHNIQUES focus on different areas of the spine. The spine can be divided into five different areas, and different schools of chiropractic focus on different parts of the spine.

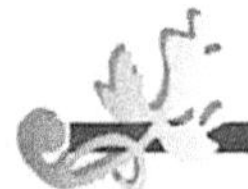

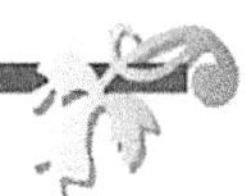

☂ Some chiropractors specialize in adjusting the two top bones in the neck. Because this area is closest to the base of the skull and the brain stem, chiropractors who focus on this area believe that misalignment in this area is much more problematic than mis-alignment in other parts of the spine.

> *Chiropractors who focus on this area believe that if this area is aligned, the rest of the spine will heal itself. Upper cervical chiropractors do not usually promote long-term chiropractic care. Instead, their goal is to get people better with the fewest adjustments possible.*

☂ Chiropractors who work on the hips, sacrum, and lower back -- the lumbar or sacral area -- have completely different beliefs. Instead of believing that the upper part of the spine is most important to health, they believe that subluxations in the lower spine affect the stability of the spine as a whole.

> *Because there are a bundle of nerve roots at the end of the spine that travel into the abdomen, organs, and legs, chiropractors who focus on the lower spine believe that subluxations here can cause neurological issues.*

☂ Some chiropractors give equal weight to the entire spine.

> *According to these chiropractors, any subluxation, no matter where it occurs on the spine, has a negative effect on the body.*

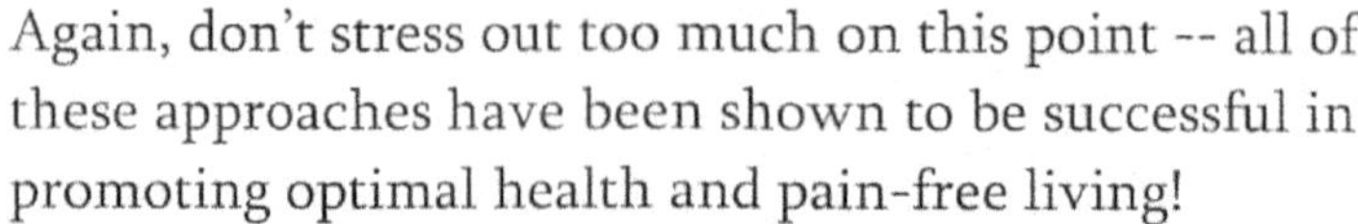

Again, don't stress out too much on this point -- all of these approaches have been shown to be successful in promoting optimal health and pain-free living!

THE USE OF FORCE

ANOTHER THING that differentiates one chiropractor from another is the amount of force they use. Different techniques require different amounts of force. While you may not need to know exactly what technique your chiropractor employs, you will most likely want to know the level of force. It is important that you are comfortable with it!

LOW-FORCE CHIROPRACTORS concentrate on trigger points, which are parts of the spine that are connected with different parts of the body. Trigger points are very sensitive, so only the smallest amount of force is needed to have an effect on the body.

> *Some chiropractors use pressure probes or wands with a very light force. Upper cervical chiropractors, those who focus on the upper neck, usually use low-force techniques as the bones in this area are smaller than the bones in the rest of the spine.*

The Logan technique is a low-force technique focused on the bottom of the spine.

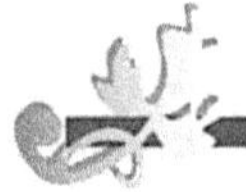

MEDIUM-FORCE CHIROPRACTIC CARE is probably the most common type of care. To understand how medium-force chiropractic works, you need to know a little bit about the idea of long or short levers. In long-lever adjustments, pressure is applied to an arm, leg, hip, or shoulder. The body is then twisted, allowing the joint being manipulated to be brought to the range of motion where it is locking up. A quick thrust moves the joint beyond that point, allowing normal range of motion to be restored. In the short-lever technique the chiropractor manipulates the vertebrae with his hands.

> *Chiropractors who use this type of technique often have their patients lie face down on a drop table. A drop table allows different parts of the body to be placed at different levels. When the chiropractor does the thrust, the table at that part of the body drops a very small amount -- less than an inch.*

HIGH-FORCE CHIROPRACTIC is pretty rare, and usually reserved for cases when a joint or bone will not be released with medium force.

> *High-force chiropractic uses the same principles as long-lever chiropractic, with more thrust applied. It is worth noting that most chiropractors prefer to use the least amount of force necessary.*

So what force is right for you?

If you want a dramatic adjustment that you can feel the results of in the office, then medium-force chiropractic is probably the way to go. If you have a low tolerance for pain or pressure, or are nervous about going to the chiropractor in the first place, a low-force adjustment is probably a good place to begin. It is important that you know that one method does not work better than another. Just because a treatment is more forceful does not mean it is working better. Whether you choose low force or medium force is rather just a matter of your preference.

You will get the same results either way.

When it comes time to make your choice, don't rush it. Do research. Ask questions. Get recommendations. Many chiropractors offer free consultations to prospective patients. We suggest that you take advantage of these to interview several chiropractors before you make your choice. By taking your time you'll be certain to find a chiropractor who suits your needs, has a philosophy you can live with, and is familiar with and has experience with your particular condition.

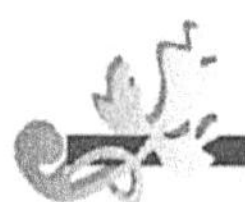

QUESTIONS TO ASK YOUR DC

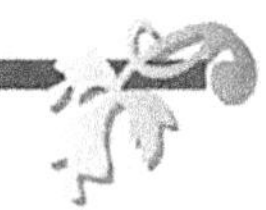

HERE ARE A FEW QUESTIONS you might want to ask your chiropractor when you first meet. If a chiropractor is not willing to spend some time answering these questions, then he or she is not for you. Move on, and work with someone who cares enough to communicate with you about your precious health!

- ♣ Do you have experience with my condition?
- ♣ Have patients with my condition improved under your care?
- ♣ How many adjustments do you estimate it will take before I feel better?
- ♣ Are you willing to treat me in conjunction with other traditional medical professionals if chiropractic treatment is not enough?
- ♣ What is your chiropractic philosophy?
- ♣ What is your chiropractic technique? Does it have a name?
- ♣ Would you describe this technique in detail?
- ♣ Would you consider yourself straight, mixing, or allopathic?
- ♣ Would you describe your technique as low force, medium force, or high force?
- ♣ Do you offer other services in addition to adjustments?
- ♣ What does a typical visit entail?

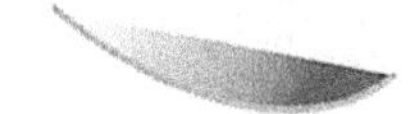

SIDEBAR: Boards Agencies Governing Chiropractic Care

THERE ARE TWO MAIN BOARDS that govern chiropractic testing and licensing. They are the Federation of Chiropractic Licensing Boards and the National Board of Chiropractic Examiners.

(1) FEDERATION OF CHIROPRACTIC LICENSING BOARDS W. 10th St., Suite 101, Greeley, CO 80634-4400; (970) 356-3500; www.fclb.org; info@fclb.org.

The mission of the Federation of Chiropractic Licensing Boards (FCLB) is "To protect the public and to serve our member boards by promoting excellence in chiropractic regulation."

Though it has been known by many different names throughout the years, the Federation of Chiropractic Licensing Boards first met in 1919, and became an official organization in 1926. The non-profit organization is dedicated to maintaining high, uniform standards in areas related to chiropractic licensure, regulation, discipline, and education.

The FCLB holds an annual conference and several district meetings, which allow issues, ideas, and viewpoints to be exchanged. At these meetings members also adopt resolutions that protect chiropractic's

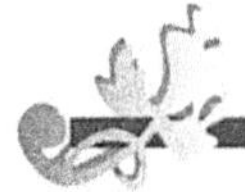

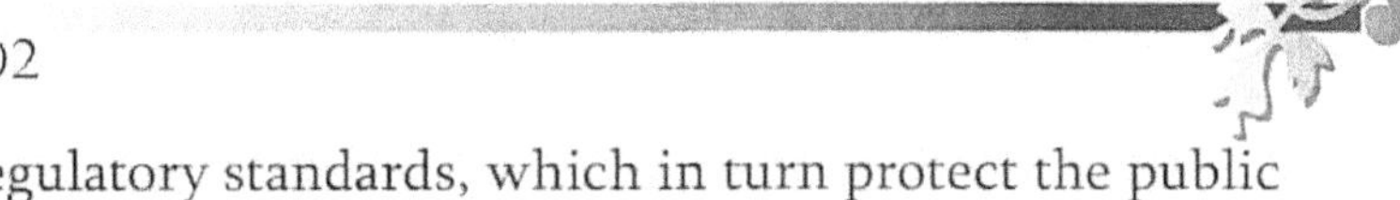

regulatory standards, which in turn protect the public using chiropractic services.

The FCLB also has a service called the CIN-BAD system, which offers databases to member boards and other subscribers. Members of the FCLB include boards which have jurisdiction to license or regulate the practice of chiropractic in the states, provinces, commonwealths, or territories of the United States, Canada, Australia, Mexico, and other countries.

(2) NATIONAL BOARD OF CHIROPRACTIC EXAMINERS, 901 54th Avenue, Greeley, CO 80634; (970) 356-9100; www.nbce.org; nbce@nbce.org.

Developed in 1963, the National Board of Chiropractic Examiners (NBCE) is a non-profit organization that provides testing programs which serve the needs of state licensing authorities, chiropractic colleges, educators and students, doctors of chiropractic, and the public.

The NBCE also develops and administers standardized national examinations according to established guidelines.

> *The goals of the organization are to promote high standards of competence, assist state licensing agencies in assessing competence, facilitate the licensure of incoming practitioners, and enhance professional credibility.*

In addition to developing and administering the tests, the NBCE also scores and reports results of different examinations. The NBCE scores are used, among other criteria, to determine whether applicants satisfy state licensing requirements.

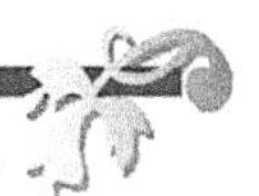

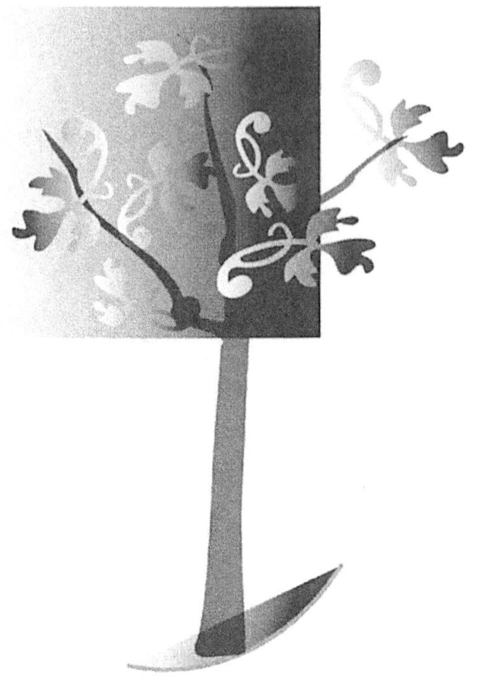

WHEN YOU BECOME a patient of a chiropractor, the first thing you'll do, before any type of treatment is administered, is have a consultation and exam.

The consultation is designed to educate the patient. Many doctors have books and articles for the patient to read and videos for the patient to watch that will give them more information about chiropractic care and what to expect.

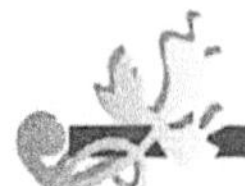

The consultation is also a great time to ask questions if you have any reservations, or just want to know a little bit more about the technique or philosophy of the chiropractor.

Before you see the doctor you'll be asked to fill out a health history form, much as you do when you go to the doctor's office. This form will ask you for information regarding the reason you are seeking treatment, general health, family health history, and lifestyle. Since it is possible for chiropractic care to treat many different health problems, it is important that you list them and talk to your chiropractor about them. Your main reason for visiting may be back pain, but wouldn't it be great if you could get your allergies under control as well?

Depending upon your chiropractor and how he does things, you may see him right away, or you may see a chiropractor's assistant trained in diagnostics. If you do see an assistant, that person's main job will be to go over your health history with you, then relay the important parts to the doctor before you see him. The assistant will probably fill you in on what to expect, and might also give you some supporting material to read or watch while you wait for the doctor.

When the doctor comes in, you can expect a battery of tests. There will be the normal tests like height, weight, and blood pressure, and there will also be tests that evaluate your spine.

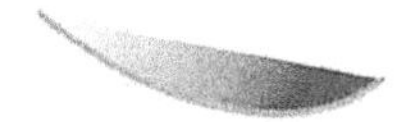

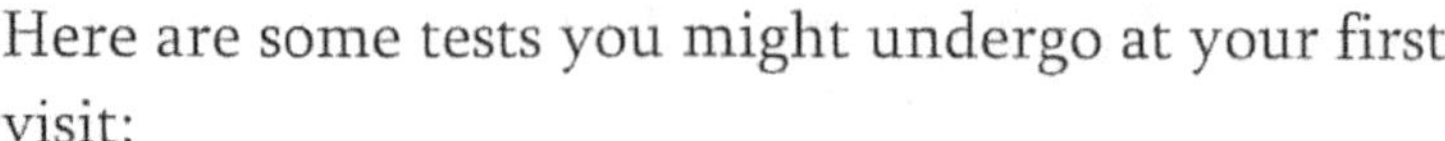

Here are some tests you might undergo at your first visit:

Visual Postural Analysis

The doctor will ask you to stand, then will assess how well you are aligned by sight. He'll look for things like whether you seem to favor a particular leg, whether one shoulder is higher than the other, whether you tilt your neck more to one side than to the other, and if your posture is straight or slouched. He may use a frame that measures variations in posture, or he may even use a high-tech machine that uses computer imaging.

Neurological Testing

This is similar to the neurological testing at your physician's office. The chiropractor will test your reflexes using a hammer. Some chiropractors run a metal pinwheel across the body to find out if any areas are numb or have decreased or increased sensitivity.

Orthopedic Testing

The chiropractor will assess the joints to see if there is any inflammation or discomfort. He or she will do this by twisting, turning, and putting pressure on certain joints. If you are there for a specific area, such as a knee, for example, the chiropractor will most likely pay particular attention to that area.

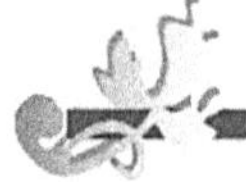

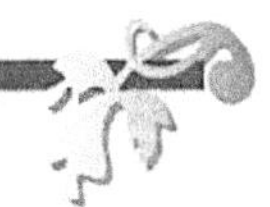

Range of Motion

In order to assess the range of motion in your joints, the doctor will ask you to bend and turn your back and neck in a particular way. Some chiropractors use a tool called a protractor to measure the range of motion.

Thermographic Testing

This tests your skin temperature, and allows the chiropractor to compare skin temperature on different parts of the body. Why is this important? Well, skin temperature is determined by blood flow to the skin. If the temperature is elevated in a particular part of body, then it indicates there is an issue there.

Motion Testing

The doctor will put his hand along your spine, then will rock it to determine its range of motion. This test will allow him to test the joints of individual vertebrae.

These are the more common tests that doctors will use to evaluate your condition, make a diagnosis, and come up with a treatment plan. Depending upon why you are at the chiropractor's office in the first place, the doctor may concentrate more on one test than another. A person who is there for neurological complaints, for example, is going to receive a different type of testing than a person who is there for elbow pain.

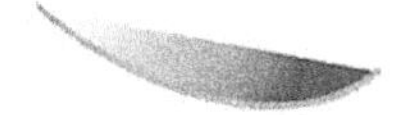

To X-Ray, Or Not To X-Ray?

MOST CHIROPRACTORS TODAY also do an x-ray of the spine. But are x-rays safe? The short answer is yes. The benefits of an x-ray far outweigh the risks.

X-rays can cause damage, but if you take the necessary precautions there is no cause for worry. Tissues that can be damaged by x-rays are usually those that reproduce quickly, like skin and the reproductive organs. Your chiropractor will make sure your reproductive organs are covered by a lead apron. It is also important to note that only a very low dose of radiation is needed to get a good image of your spine, and that x-ray testing is subject to very strict health and safety regulations that protect both the person getting the x-ray, and the person giving it.

Will your chiropractor take an x-ray?

Well, it really depends on his philosophy. Some doctors don't believe that subluxations show up on x-rays, while others do. But if you want a precise adjustment, an x-ray is the way to go.

A chiropractor may take an x-ray of your entire spine, or he may concentrate on just one area. The x-ray will not only help in your diagnosis, it will also determine your treatment.

Once a diagnosis is made, your chiropractor will discuss treatment options with you. He will most

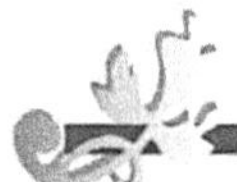

likely go over why you have your condition, what it is going to take to resolve it, how many treatments you will need, and what you can expect in terms of recovery. He'll probably tell you exactly what areas of the spine are being impinged and which vertebrae are being affected. The doctor may also suggest other treatments to support your overall health. Most chiropractors do not do adjustments on the first visit.

SUBSEQUENT VISITS

AFTER YOUR INITIAL CONSULTATION, you can expect an adjustment at your next visit. In all likelihood, your chiropractor has come up with a treatment plan that details how many adjustments you will receive during the particular course of your treatment.

How often will you have to go?

That really depends. If you are seeking chiropractic as a form of health maintenance, you'll probably need to visit only once every two or three months. If you are going for a particular complaint -- pain or injury, for example -- you might start off at three times per week for a couple of weeks, and then gradually start to taper off.

What is an adjustment like?

Well, that really depends upon your chiropractor's technique and the amount of force he uses. As mentioned before, there are almost 50 different schools of chiropractic, and each of them adjusts in a somewhat unique way. However, there are certain things that you can expect.

Depending upon your chiropractor's office, you may be treated in a private room, or you may be treated in a larger room that accommodates several patients at once.

The chiropractor should explain everything as he or she goes along. If he is using a drop table, ask him to show you how it works. The chiropractor should

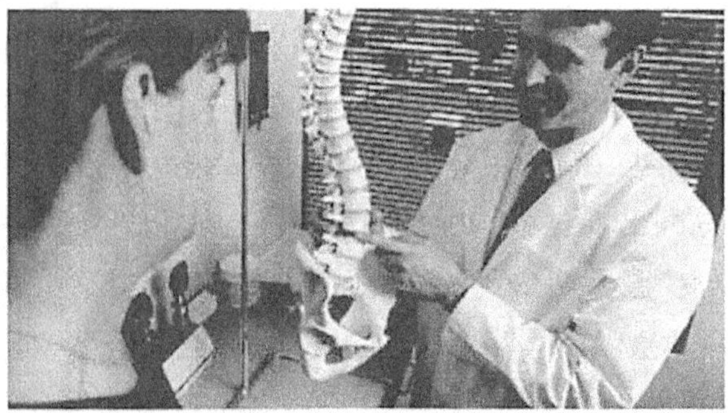

demonstrate the amount of pressure he will be using so you won't be surprised. And don't worry, your chiropractor will not sneak up on you and adjust! He will tell you before he makes the adjustment. If things have been well explained there is no reason to be tense, so relax! If you still feel nervous, perhaps there are a few questions you would still like to ask. Take your time and ask them. Your chiropractor should be happy to answer them.

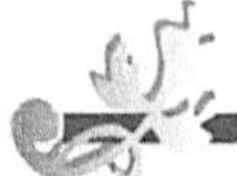

Chapter 6: The Adjustment

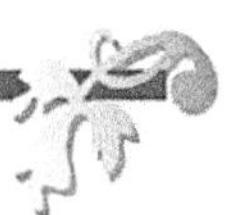

In most cases, the adjustment will be so gentle that you won't even be aware that it has occurred! It is not uncommon for recently adjusted patients to say, *"Is that it?"* In cases where joints are really locked a little more force might be in order. The patient might feel a little more thrust and might even hear a popping sound. Don't worry! This isn't dangerous! The popping sound is very similar to what happens when you crack your knuckles -- gas is being released in the joints as they move. There should not be any pain involved in an adjustment. If there is pain, tell your chiropractor right away.

So what happens after an adjustment? Will you feel the effects right away?

About 40 to 45 percent of chiropractic patients feel some relief immediately following an adjustment. Another 50 percent don't feel much different at all. Remember -- your chiropractor has prescribed a course of treatment for you, and it will most likely take the whole course of treatment for you to experience significant improvement. About 5 percent of people will actually be a little sore or stiff the day following treatment. This is normal! As the spine is being aligned, those muscles and soft tissues that have been being used incorrectly now have to get used to their new, and better, position!

About how long will it take you to restore your body to its full function?

Well, that depends on the state of your body when you walked into the chiropractor's office! But just as it takes a lot longer to build something than it does to tear it down, restoring your health is going to take some time.

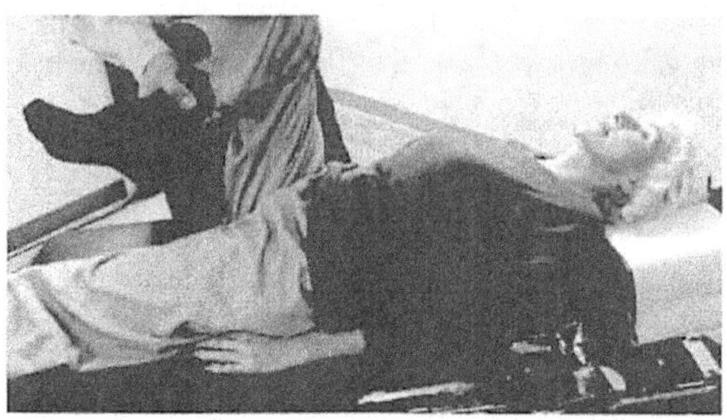

There are a few rules of thumb that can help you determine how long a haul you are in for. Your chiropractor is the best person to ask, and he should have a good estimate. But generally, the better the condition of the spine, the faster you are going to recover. This is why children, whose spines are relatively malleable and not yet permanently damaged, can recover more quickly than adults. If there is damage to the soft tissues and even degeneration of bone as a result of misuse, you can expect a year or two of treatment to restore as much function as possible. If you are a senior it may take even longer. And while all damage can't be reversed by chiropractic care, chiropractic care can certainly improve the body's health and function.

> *Chiropractic is not a quick fix -- it's a choice in lifestyle just like eating well and exercising. You take care of your teeth by regularly going to the dentist. You have a yearly physical to make sure your health is in good order. Well, don't forget to*

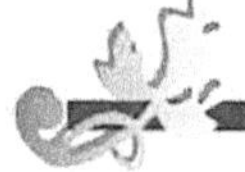

Chapter 6: The Adjustment

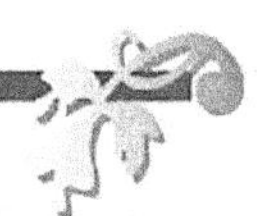

take regular care of your spine and nervous system! With regular chiropractic care you can live life to the fullest! You can experience greater mobility, more flexibility, increased vitality, and less pain and illness. You can help your body help to heal itself, and give it the gift of optimal health.

SIDEBAR: Chiropractic Research

HERE ARE JUST A FEW of the more recent studies that show how effective and safe chiropractic care is. The condition is listed, followed by the study's findings. For more studies go to the web site of the Foundation for Chiropractic Education and Research (FCER).

For Acute and Chronic Pain

"Patients with chronic low-back pain treated by chiropractors showed greater improvement and satisfaction at one month than patients treated by family physicians. Satisfaction scores were higher for chiropractic patients. A higher proportion of chiropractic patients (56 percent vs. 13 percent) reported that their low-back pain was better or much better, whereas nearly one-third of medical patients reported their low-back pain was worse or much worse."

Nyiendo et al (2000), Journal of Manipulative and Physiological Therapeutics

"In a randomized controlled trial, 183 patients with neck pain were randomly allocated to manual therapy (spinal mobilization), physiotherapy (mainly exercise), or general practitioner care (counseling, education, and drugs) in a 52-week study. The clinical outcomes measured showed that manual therapy resulted in faster recovery than physiotherapy and general practitioner care. Moreover, total costs of the manual therapy-treated patients were about one-third of the costs of physiotherapy or general practitioner care."

Korthals-de Bos et al (2003), British Medical Journal

✌ In Comparison to Other Treatment Alternatives

"Acute and chronic chiropractic patients experienced better outcomes in pain, functional disability, and patient satisfaction; clinically important differences in pain and disability improvement were found for chronic patients."

Haas et al (2005), Journal of Manipulative and Physiological Therapeutics

"In our randomized, controlled trial, we compared the effectiveness of manual therapy, physical therapy, and continued care by a general practitioner in patients with non specific neck pain. The success rate at seven weeks was twice as high

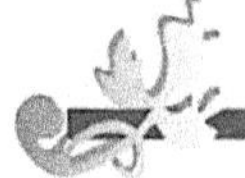

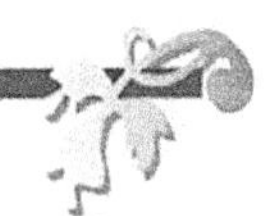

for the manual therapy group (68.3 percent) as for the continued care group (general practitioner). Manual therapy scored better than physical therapy on all outcome measures. Patients receiving manual therapy had fewer absences from work than patients receiving physical therapy or continued care, and manual therapy and physical therapy each resulted in statistically significant less analgesic use than continued care."

Hoving et al (2002), Annals of Internal Medicine

For Headaches

"Cervical spine manipulation was associated with significant improvement in headache outcomes in trials involving patients with neck pain and/or neck dysfunction and headache."

McCrory, Penzlen, Hasselblad, Gray (2001), Duke Evidence Report

"The results of this study show that spinal manipulative therapy is an effective treatment for tension headaches... four weeks after cessation of treatment... the patients who received spinal manipulative therapy experienced a sustained therapeutic benefit in all major outcomes in contrast to the patients that received amitriptyline therapy, who reverted to baseline values."

Boline et al (1995), Journal of Manipulative and Physiological Therapeutics

✍ Cost Effectiveness

"Chiropractic care appeared relatively cost-effective for the treatment of chronic low-back pain. Chiropractic and medical care performed comparably for acute patients. Practice-based clinical outcomes were consistent with systematic reviews of spinal manipulative efficacy: manipulation-based therapy is at least as good as and, in some cases, better than other therapeusis."

Haas et al (2005), Journal of Manipulative and Physiological Therapeutics

✍ Patient Satisfaction

"Chiropractic patients were found to be more satisfied with their back care providers after four weeks of treatment than were medical patients. Results from observational studies suggested that back pain patients are more satisfied with chiropractic care than with medical care. Additionally, studies conclude that patients are more satisfied with chiropractic care than they were with physical therapy after six weeks."

Hertzman-Miller et al (2002), American Journal of Public Health

✍ Popularity of Chiropractic

"Chiropractic is the largest, most regulated, and best recognized of the complementary and

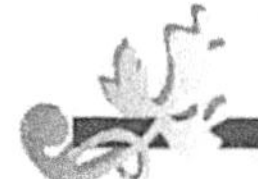

alternative medicine (CAM) professions. CAM patient surveys show that chiropractors are used more often than any other alternative provider group, and patient satisfaction with chiropractic care is very high. There is steadily increasing patient use of chiropractic in the United States, which has tripled in the past two decades."

Meeker, Haldeman (2002), Annals of InternaMedicine

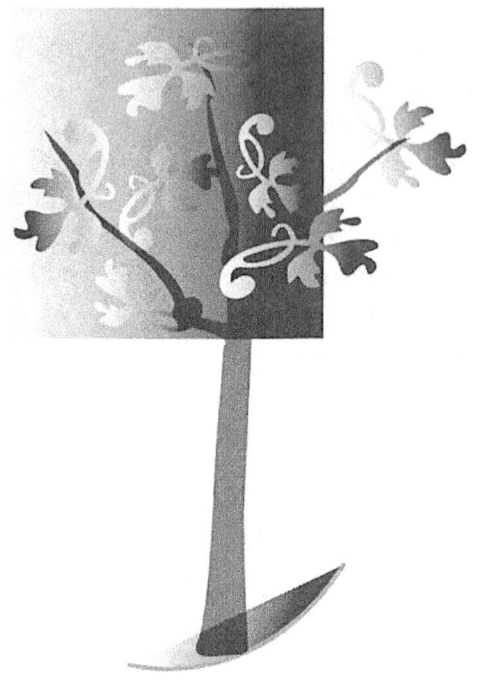

DURING ITS HUNDRED-YEAR history chiropractic care has had to constantly refute a small but powerful handful of myths, deal with the force of conventional medicine, and try to turn skeptics around. But guess what? Despite all that, chiropractic is the second-largest health care system in America, and the largest drug-free healing profession in the world. Wow!

CHAPTER
7

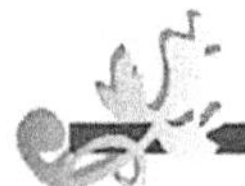

As a matter of fact, in the last few years there have been some studies and surveys done that have looked at the current status of chiropractic, have gauged the public's attitude toward the profession, and have forecasted the future of the profession. And it looks like chiropractic is here to stay!

In July of 1998, the findings of a very comprehensive study regarding chiropractic was released by the Institute for Alternative Futures. Among the findings was the fact that the number of chiropractors could reach 103,000 by the year 2010. Considering that there were only 55,000 chiropractors when the study was done in 1998, that's a huge increase! Another study, this one done by the American Journal of Public Health, reported that the number of chiropractors and the percent of the population using chiropractic care has doubled during the last 15 to 20 years.

> *As the growth of chiropractic care increases, so does the number of graduates coming out of chiropractic colleges. It is estimated that by the year 2010, 5,000 new chiropractors will graduate per year!*

Why is chiropractic care continuing to become more popular?

Well, part of chiropractic's success is due to the shift in models of health care. Improving the function and quality of one's life is becoming just as important -- and sometimes more so -- as treating specific disease

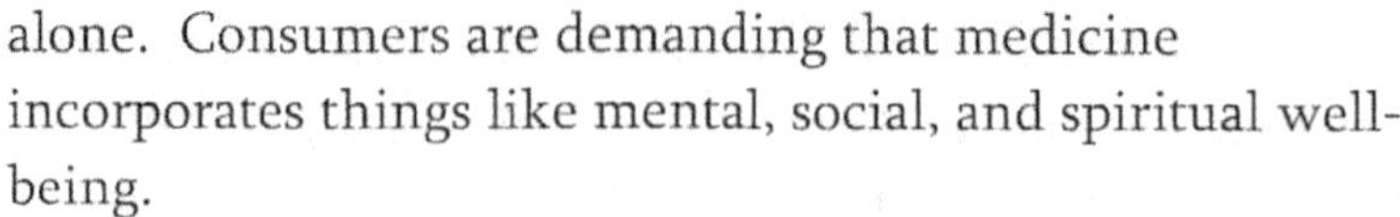

alone. Consumers are demanding that medicine incorporates things like mental, social, and spiritual well-being.

> *The focus today is not so much on curing disease and illness as it is on preventing it. In fact, a survey done by the Journal of the American Medical Association showed that 42 percent of Americans used alternative care because "the treatment promotes health rather than just focusing on illness."*

Just consider what newest all-time homerun king Barry Bonds has to say about chiropractic.

> *"I hurt my back swinging the bat... our trainer recommended that I try chiropractic. At first, I was skeptical, but after seeing a lot of the players on the team using it, I thought I would give it a try... I knew I had to get some more of that."*[5]

Evander Holyfield, former World Heavy-weight Boxing Champion, raves in the very same fashion.

> *"I found that going to a chiropractor helps my performance. Once I drove 20 miles to see a chiropractor before a flight. I have to have my adjustment before I go into the ring."*[6]

But the fans of chiropractic are not limited to the world of sports. Celebrities such as Demi Moore, Kim Bassinger, Denzel Washington, Mel Gibson, Arnold Schwarzenegger, and many more reap the rewards of chiropractic to stay looking and feeling their very best.

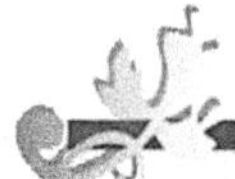

People of today have a certain demand when it comes to wellness. Just check out the throngs of people flocking to the gym to maintain good health and stave off disease and illness. These same folks are open to using alternative therapies such as chiropractic care to prevent future illness and to maintain health and vitality.

In fact, in a study done by the Journal of the American Medical Association, it was found that there were 243 million more visits to alternative providers than there were to all types of traditional primary care physicians combined in United States!

CHIROPRACTIC: MYTH VS. REALITY

Chiropractic treatments hurt.

MYTH. Most patients find adjustments very relieving. Occasionally, there may be some minor discomfort, which would not be described as "painful" and does not last more than 12 to 48 hours.

The "pop" that patients sometimes hear while being adjusted is the release of gas bubbles that have become trapped in the joint. It's the same as when you "crack" your knuckles and can provide a similar sensation of release. The loudness of the sound varies from patient to patient and has very little or no meaning.

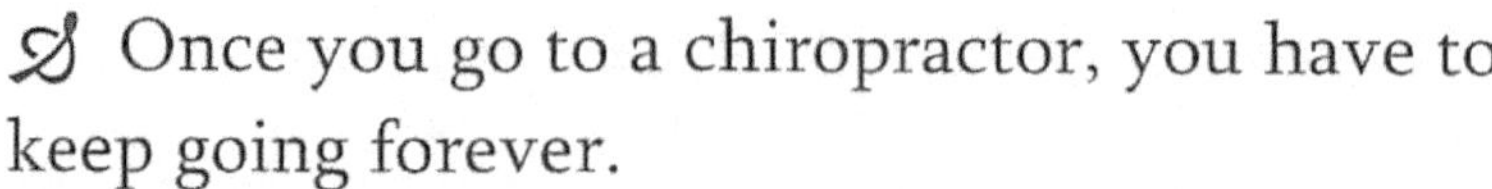

Once you go to a chiropractor, you have to keep going forever.

MYTH. Many patients choose to continue their chiropractic visits simply because of the incredible health and vitality they've discovered chiropractic care brings them.

> *Chiropractors provide three general levels of treatment and the patient ultimately chooses which best fits their needs.*

Chiropractic care is not safe.

MYTH. Since chiropractic medicine seeks to restore your body to its natural state of health, unlike traditional medicine which seeks to alter your body via medications and/or surgery, chiropractic is recognized as one of the safest types of health care in the world! It does not include any of the nasty side effects or risks associated with drug therapy or surgery.

> In fact, that is why chiropractors enjoy the lowest malpractice rates in the entire field of medicine! So even the insurance companies have been forced to admit there is no safer care for you and your back pain than chiropractic care!

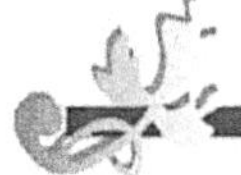

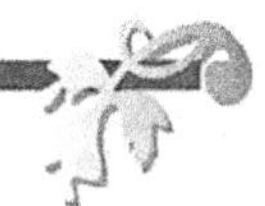

✍ You need a referral from your primary care physician before you can see a chiropractor.

MYTH. You do not need a referral from your family doctor or primary care physician before visiting a chiropractor.

> *A fact which is unknown to most people is that federal and state regulations view chiropractors as a first contact physician -- in other words, they ARE primary care physicians!*

✍ Chiropractic care is expensive.

MYTH. First off, the majority of all insured American workers have coverage for chiropractic care, and that percentage is increasingly regularly. In addition, most doctors offer affordable payment plans to accommodate those who are not covered.

If you happen to have to pay out-of-pocket, you can rest assured you'll still be saving money over the alternative. Just consider what Met Life Insurance has to say about the cost of chiropractic care versus the surgical alternative:

> *"The average "medical non-surgical back" costs $7,210, and the average "surgical back" costs $13,990. But according to research from the North Carolina Back Pain Institute, the average chiropractic case costs approximately $800 for the same diagnostic code."* [7]

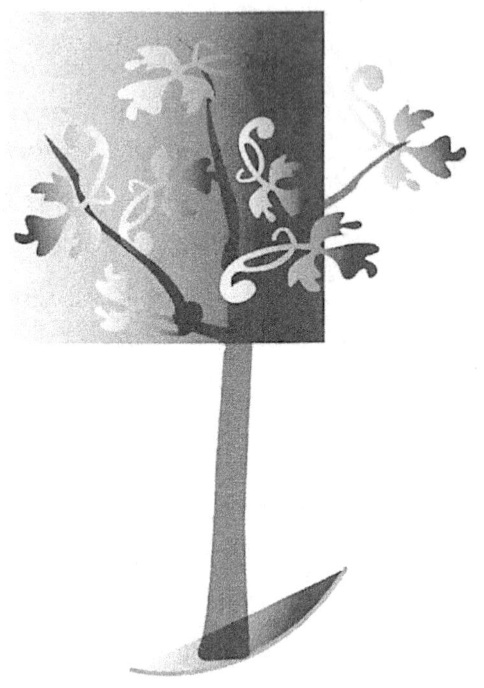

Understanding The Language Of Chiropractic

DEPENDING UPON your chiropractor, his philosophy, technique, and school, you may hear some of these terms around the office. This handy guide should help you know exactly what your chiropractor is talking about! If your chiropractor uses a word that you don't know or understand, ask him for an explanation.

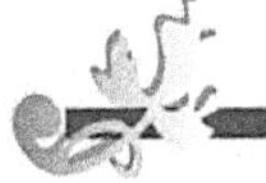

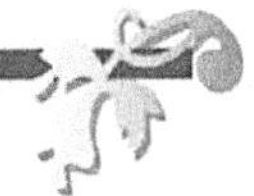

- ♣ Activator Adjusting Instrument. A handheld instrument used by chiropractors who assert that slightly misaligned vertebrae can be tapped back into place with a mallet.

- ♣ Acute back pain. Back pain that lasts a short while, usually a few days to several weeks. Episodes lasting longer than three months are not considered acute.

- ♣ Atlas. Uppermost vertebra of the neck.

- ♣ Atlas orthogonal technique (A.O.T.). One of many methods of correcting cervical "subluxations" claimed to be responsible for problems anywhere in the body.

- ♣ Atlas subluxation complex (ASC). An alleged entity that some chiropractors feel is the most common and the most serious vertebral misalignment. Chiropractors who practice specific "upper cervical techniques" focus on the ASC.

- ♣ Barge analysis. A contemporary technique, developed by a straight chiropractor, used to locate alleged shifting of a disk nucleus said to cause tortipelvis/torticollis, spinal distortions, or curvatures. Rotation of a spinous process toward the wide side of a disk space on the concave side of a spinal curve (the opposite of what is normally seen) is thought to indicate that the disk is improperly centered.

- ♣ Bio Energetic Synchronization Technique (B.E.S.T.). A method that involves measuring leg length to determine whether "imbalances" exist in the

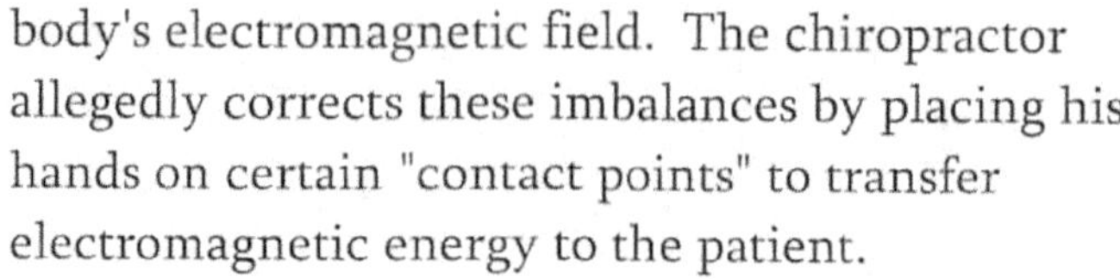

body's electromagnetic field. The chiropractor allegedly corrects these imbalances by placing his hands on certain "contact points" to transfer electromagnetic energy to the patient.

- ♣ Bio-kinetics. A new technique in which a special adjustment with an instrument is made between the atlas and the skull to relieve dozens of ailments ranging from asthma to psoriasis. This cure-all spinal adjustment corrects subluxations and "reconstructs the spine."

- ♣ Blair upper cervical technique. Another technique that concentrates upon correction of vertebral misalignments at the top of the neck as a method of removing nerve interference in the spine.

- ♣ C.A. Abbreviation for "chiropractic assistant."

- ♣ Carver technique. Method developed by Willard Carver, an early Palmer student who formulated his own theories about subluxations and nerve interference. He the Carver Chiropractic college in 1908. Carver developed a technique in which traction and pressure are applied to the spine just before making a manual thrust. This is called the "Tracto-Thrust" system.

- ♣ Cavitation. The "pop" that occurs in a spinal joint when vertebral surfaces (facets) are separated to create a vacuum that pulls in nitrogen gas.

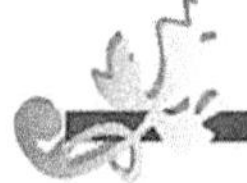

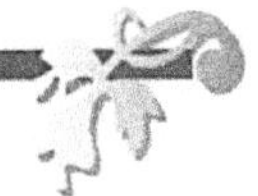

- Cervical vertebrae. There are seven vertebrae in the cervical or neck area of the spine.

- Chiropractic Biophysics (CBP). Method of chiropractic analysis and treatment in which spinal corrections are based on theoretical calculations related to posture and spinal curvature. This technique advocates adjustments, traction, and exercises intended to develop "normal" neck and low-back curvature.

- Chronic back pain. Back pain episode that lasts more than three months.

- Contact Reflex Analysis (CRA). A testing procedure in which diagnoses are made by testing muscle strength while placing manual pressure on alleged "reflex points." The results are then used to prescribe vitamin supplements and/or homeopathic products. Cox flexion-distraction technique. Method of applying manually controlled distraction or stretching to specific spinal segments with the assistance of a movable table. Not a manipulation technique.

- D.C. Abbreviation for "doctor of chiropractic."

- D.C.M. (Doctor of Chiropractic Medicine). New degree being considered by at least one chiropractic college, which believes that some form of drug therapy may be appropriate for a properly specialized chiropractic practice.

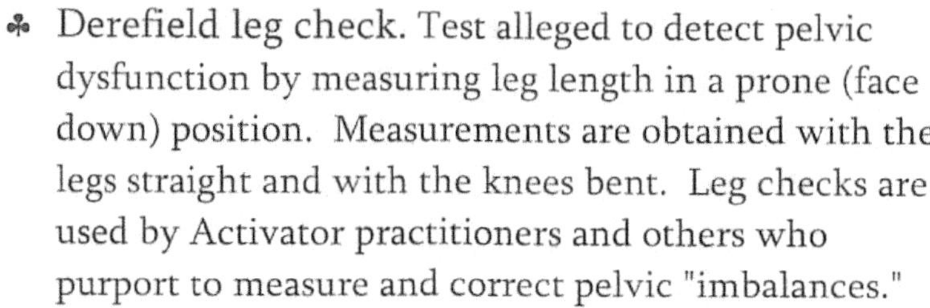

- Derefield leg check. Test alleged to detect pelvic dysfunction by measuring leg length in a prone (face down) position. Measurements are obtained with the legs straight and with the knees bent. Leg checks are used by Activator practitioners and others who purport to measure and correct pelvic "imbalances."

- Directional nonforce technique (DNFT). Method of diagnosing and correcting subluxations by applying thumb pressure to the spine and checking leg length, which supposedly changes when correction is made.

- Dynamic thrust. Chiropractic adjustment delivered suddenly and forcefully to move vertebrae, often resulting in a popping sound.

- Flexion-distraction technique. Useful method of stretching the spine with the patient in a face down position on a table that allows manually applied flexion and traction to be applied to specific spinal segments.

- Full-spine technique. Method of adjusting or manipulating any of the vertebrae from the neck down.

- Gonstead technique. System of correcting pelvic and sacral subluxations to correct secondary subluxations elsewhere in the spine. The alleged problem areas are located by motion palpation and skin-temperature instrument measurement and confirmed with full-spine x-ray examination.

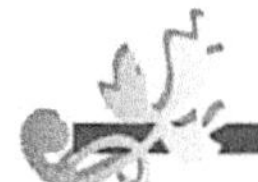

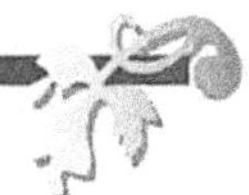

- Grostic procedure. Upper cervical technique that depends upon x-ray examination to measure and detect misalignments between the atlas and the skull. Thea Adjustment can be made with an instrument or be done manually by placing pressure on the side of the neck at the base of the skull.

- Hole-in-One (H.I.O.). Method of adjusting the atlas (the topmost vertebra at the base of the skull). Proponents claim that this will improve health and facilitate correction of subluxations elsewhere in the spine.

- Innate Intelligence. An alleged inborn ability of the body to heal itself, which chiropractors believe is enhanced by spinal adjustments.

- Intervertebral disk. The tough cartilage that serves as a cushion between two vertebrae.

- Kale method. Variety of upper cervical adjustment in which a "toggle adjustment," or a sudden, shallow thrust is applied to the side of the neck to correct atlas subluxations, often with the patient in a knee-chest position on a special table.

- Leander's method. Method that utilizes a motorized table for loosening or mobilizing the spine with flexion-distraction-type stretching before a spinal adjustment.

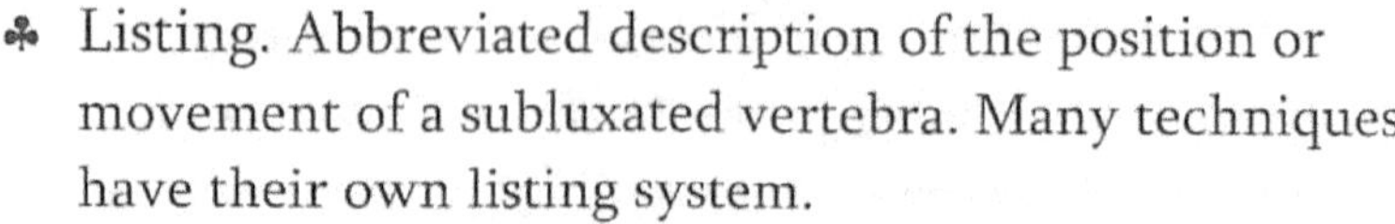

- ♣ Listing. Abbreviated description of the position or movement of a subluxated vertebra. Many techniques have their own listing system.

- ♣ Locked spinal joint. Sudden binding that occurs when two joint surfaces are shifted out of their normal alignment by an awkward movement that triggers muscle spasm. The result may also be called an "acute locked back."

- ♣ Logan method. A non-thrusting method in which thumb pressure is used to correct alleged sacral subluxations and leg deficiency, claimed to affect the entire spine.

- ♣ Long-lever manipulation. Method of spinal manipulation in which a general technique is used to stretch or loosen several vertebrae at a time.

- ♣ Lumbar vertebrae. The five bones in the lower-back portion of the spine.

- ♣ Lumbo-pelvic techniques. Technique used to adjust any "manipulative lesion" in the joints of the lumbar spine and pelvis. Lumbo-pelvic "distortions" are attributed to postural alterations, leg-length inequality, tilting of the lumbar vertebrae, loss of mobility, and other "lesions" that require manipulation of the pelvis and lower back. Leg-length testing is often used to detect lumbo-pelvic distortions.

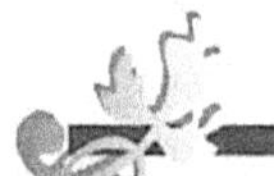

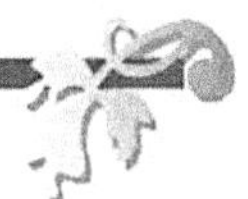

* Lumbosacral strain. Strain or injury of joints or ligaments at the base of the spine where the last lumbar vertebra (L5) is connected to the sacrum. Strain or disk degeneration in this area is probably the most common cause of low-back pain.

* Maintenance care. Subluxation-based program of periodic spinal examinations and "adjustments" alleged to help maintain the patient's health.

* Meric system. Chiropractic system based on the theory that specific spinal joints are associated with specific organs, requiring adjustment of certain vertebrae for certain diseases.

* "Mixer." Chiropractor who uses physical therapy and other natural treatment methods in addition to manual manipulation of the spine.

* Mobilization. Method of manipulation, movement, or stretching to increase range of motion in muscles and joints that does not involve a high-velocity thrust.

* Motion palpation. Useful method of locating fixations and loss of mobility in the spine by feeling the motion of specific spinal segments as the patient moves.

* Musculoskeletal. Referring to structures involving tendons, muscles, ligaments, and joints.

* Nerve root. One of the two nerve bundles emerging from the spinal cord that join to form a segmental spinal nerve.

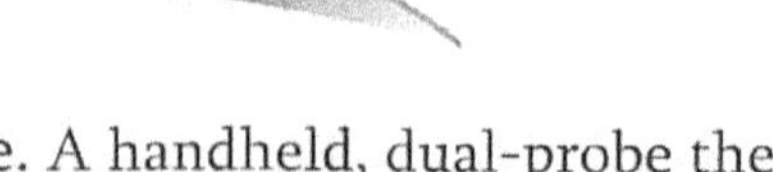

- **Nervo-Scope.** A handheld, dual-probe thermocouple gadget purported to locate "subluxations" by measuring skin temperature on both sides of the spine.

- **Nimmo method.** Technique that uses digital pressure on trigger points to relax muscles said to be pulling vertebrae out of alignment.

- **Nonforce techniques.** Various reflex techniques and muscle-treatment methods that do not involve forceful manipulation.

- **Objective straight chiropractors.** Chiropractors whose sole objective is to "correct vertebral subluxations -- not because they cause disease or are associated with any medical condition, but simply because the body works better without them . . . . and that alone justifies their correction."

- **Orthogonal methods.** Upper cervical measurements and techniques that often require use of instruments and machines to correct what are claimed to be minute but all-important subluxations of the atlas.

- **Pettibone method.** Upper cervical adjustive technique that utilizes an instrument to adjust the atlas. Orthogonal lines are used to measure the full spine.

- **P.I.** Abbreviation for "personal injury." Used in the phrases "PI practice" and "PI seminar," which focus on patients with occupational or auto injuries.

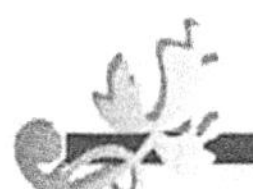

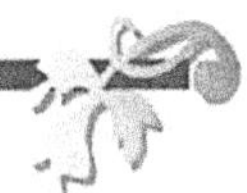

* Pierce-Stillwagon method. Technique similar to
  Sacro-Occipital Technique which involves contacts
  and other maneuvers applied to cervical and pelvic
  areas to produce effects in remote muscles, organs,
  and joints. A full-spine x-ray examination is
  considered essential for pelvic analysis. Uses a heat-
  detecting instrument (Derma Therm-O-Graph) to
  monitor subluxation correction.

* Sacro-Occiptal Technique. Pseudoscientific
  diagnostic and treatment method said to involve
  analysis and correction of sacral and cranial
  distortions to improve circulation of cerebrospinal
  fluid. The degree of alleged correction obtained is
  monitored by checking leg length.

* Sacrum. The triangular bone that serves as a base for
  the spinal column and connects the pelvic bones.

* Short-lever manipulation. A method of spinal
  manipulation in which contact is made on a vertebral
  process to move a single vertebra.

* SMT. An abbreviation for "spinal manipulative
  therapy."

* Spinal adjustment. A chiropractic term that most
  chiropractors use to describe whatever method(s) they
  use to correct spinal problems, whether by hand or
  with an instrument.

* Spinal manipulation. A forceful, high-velocity thrust
  that stretches a joint beyond its passive range of

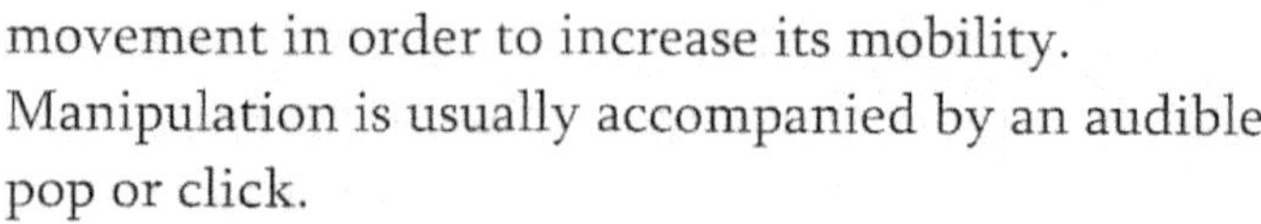

movement in order to increase its mobility. Manipulation is usually accompanied by an audible pop or click.

♣ Straight chiropractor. A chiropractor who believes in chiropractic's original doctrine that most health problems are caused by misaligned spinal bones ("vertebral subluxations") and are correctable by manual manipulation of the spine.

♣ Subluxation. The medical definition is "incomplete or partial dislocation"-- a condition visible on x-ray films, in which the bony surfaces of a joint no longer face each other exactly but remain partially aligned.

♣ Sweat method. Atlas orthogonal technique in which the atlas is adjusted using a special table and a solenoid stylus placed against the side of the neck just behind and below the ear.

♣ Thermography. A diagnostic procedure that images heat from body surfaces. Commonly used by chiropractors but not found to be effective in locating pinched nerves or subluxated vertebrae.

♣ Thompson terminal point technique. A chiropractic adjustment performed on a table in which the supporting cushions drop an inch or two when a thrust is applied to the spine. Practitioners locate subluxations by checking leg lengths with the legs straight, the knees bent, or the head turned to either side.

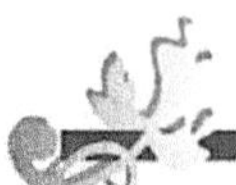

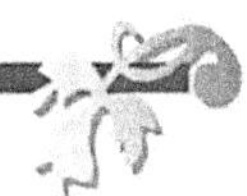

- Thoracic vertebrae. There are twelve vertebrae in the thoracic or upper-back portion of the spine.

- Toggle recoil technique. Manipulation performed with a sudden shallow thrust (toggle) followed by quick withdrawal (recoil) of the chiropractor's hands while the patient is relaxed.

- Total body modification (T.B.M.). Method that involves locating stressed organs or body areas so that "tried and tested reflex points and muscle testing" can be used to stimulate specific areas of the spine.

- Upper cervical specific. Technique that uses a number of specific chiropractic adjustments designed to correct atlas and upper cervical subluxations.

- Vax-D (vertebral axial decompression). A form of traction using a device that stretches and releases the spine while the patient lies face down.

- Vertebra. Bony segment of the spine that encircles and helps protect the spinal cord and nerves. The plural of vertebra is vertebrae.

- Vertebral artery. Arteries, one on each side, that thread through holes in the six upper cervical vertebrae.

- Vertebral subluxation complex. A modern chiropractic term for the chiropractic subluxation.

FOOTNOTES

[1] *Journal of American Medical Association* (Jan 22/29, 1997, Vol. 277, p. 301-306)

[2] *American Journal of Neuroradiol* (April 1999, 20:697-705)

[3] *American Society of Health-System Pharmacists: Injectable Corticosteroid Suspensions Products-description*, 28 February 2006

[4] *Ah, My Aching Back! Back Pain Treatments Can Be Tailor-Made* -- NPR (Morning Edition -- March 9, 2006)

[5] *Dynamic Chiropractic* (Oct. 22, 2001)

[6] *Today's Chiropractic Magazine* (December 1998 issue)

[7] *Carey TS, et al. The outcomes and costs of care for acute low back pain among patients seen by primary care practitioners, chiropractors and orthopedic surgeons.* New England Journal of Medicine (1995;333:913-17)

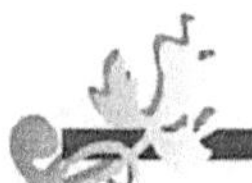

THE *Healthy* ALTERNATIVE

Why Chiropractic Care Is the Safest and Most Effective Way to Restore and Maintain Optimal Health...Naturally!

"The one book that will forever change the way people stop their pain and recapture the health of their youth… naturally!"

Here's what you'll discover in the pages of *The Healthy Alternative*:

- Why chiropractic care is the best way to stop your pain and regain your health when you're not willing to risk suffering the dangerous side effects of drugs or surgery.

- How chiropractic care can extend and improve your life and the lives of your loved ones.

- Why thousands of people are raving about how chiropractic care has finally allowed them to "feel good"!

- The TRUTH about chiropractic care what the "Medical Community" doesn't want you to know and will never tell you about chiropractic care.

- ...and much more about achieving and maintaining optimal health... naturally!

"Anybody who's truly looking for the answer to health and wellness, naturally, without the use of harmful substances or wacky medical treatments MUST read **The Healthy Alternative**. It dispels some of the ridiculous myths about chiropractic care and really tells readers exactly what they can do to eliminate their pain and recapture their vitality… naturally. It's a must read!"

—Todd Brown
CCN, Board Certified Clinical Nutritionist

"I've had literally dozens of chiropractic treatments and even have an uncle and a close friend who are chiropractors. However, it wasn't until I read *The Healthy Alternative* that I truly understood how chiropractic actually transforms your body from the inside out! It's no wonder that so many people are discovering that chiropractic care can be their newfound fountain of youth. It's getting them to look better and feel younger than they have in years. Give this book a good read and you'll be as amazed as I was!"

—Damian Lanfranchi
Author and Editor of *The Instant Chiropractic Newsletter*

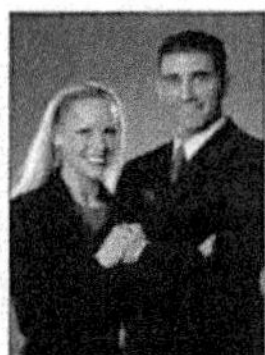

Dr. Mike was born and raised in Western New York. He enjoys spending time with his family and friends. He also has a passion for traveling to exotic locations and learning about new cultures. He had his career goals planned from a young age, and promptly began achieving them after graduation. He moved to Atlanta, Georgia where he studied physical therapy and received his accredited certification in physiological therapeutics. He then moved to St. Louis and received his 2nd bachelor degree in Life Sciences and finally his Doctorate from the prestigious Logan University in St. Louis, MO. Dr. Fair fast tracked her undergraduate studies in Biology and graduated Magna Cum Laude from Gannon University with her Bachelor's degree in three years. She graduated Cum Laude from the prestigious Logan University. While at Logan, she was also honored with several awards such as Health Care Achievement Award and a National Leadership Award. Dr. Fair has a Fellowship in Pediatrics and Peri-natal care from the International Chiropractic Pediatric Association. Dr. Fair and Dr. Gambacorta married after graduation and they now have two wonderful little boys, Michael and Alexander, as well as a house full of animals. They spend their family time traveling, going on new adventures, and playing outdoors. They are fulfilling their life-long mission of helping people and changing lives through their practice.

Dr Michael & Dr Torri Gambacorta

www.ingramcontent.com/pod-product-compliance
Lightning Source LLC
Chambersburg PA
CBHW072236150726
48002CB00005B/2125